Sue Dengate is a psychology gradu

teacher. As a result of her own

became a food intolerance counse

effects of foods on children's heal.

Her research concerning behavioural effects of a common bread
preservative was the first study of this topic ever published in a
medical journal. In 2001 she completed a 'supermarket tour'
around the world, checking food additive use in fifteen countries. Her first three books, *Different Kids*, *Fed Up* and *The
Failsafe Cookbook*, are bestsellers. She runs a support website
at www.fedupwithfoodadditives.info.

Also by Sue Dengate

Different Kids
Fed Up
The Failsafe Cookbook

Fed Up
with
Asthma

**How food affects asthma and
what you can do about it**

Sue Dengate

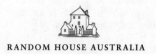

RANDOM HOUSE AUSTRALIA

Random House Australia Pty Ltd
20 Alfred Street, Milsons Point, NSW 2061
http://www.randomhouse.com.au

Sydney   New York   Toronto
London   Auckland   Johannesburg

First published by Random House Australia 2003

National Library of Australia
Cataloguing-in-Publication Entry

Dengate, Sue, 1948– .
Fed up with asthma : how food affects asthma and what you
can do about it.

Includes index.
ISBN 1 74051 056 9.

1. Asthma – Diet therapy. 2. Asthma – Prevention. 3. Food additives – Health
aspects. I. Title

616.2380654

Cover photograph by Getty images
Illustrations by Joanne Van Os
Typeset in 11/13 pt Times by Midland Typesetters, Maryborough, Victoria
Printed and bound by Griffin Press, Netley, South Australia

10 9 8 7 6 5 4 3 2 1

Acknowledgements

Many people contributed to this book in various ways. I am particularly indebted to the team at Asthma NT: former executive officer Brian McCarthy, current executive officer Michelle Menzies, asthma educators Naomi Rosenberg and especially Jan Saunders; librarian Helen Edney at the Northern Territory Reference Library, lactation consultant Clare Affleck; and Deborah Halliwell.

Grateful thanks, also, to those who have shared their experiences and ideas with me (some names have been changed in the actual stories to protect privacy): Sue Armstrong, Cathy Bannister, Moya Connell, Heather Curdie, Nancy Devlin, Julie Gilfoyle, Brigid Goodman, Judy Horner, Gillian Helyar, Brenda Hunting, Jill and Richard Newton, Jane Moore, Christine Orman, Heather Perry, Jenny Saal, Peter Saunders, Stephanie Stevens, Bernard and Marie Trudgett, Erica Waite, Rick Williams and Roxana Woodward.

I am obliged to the many members of the Food Intolerance Network who have written to discuss asthma and the effects of food—you have contributed greatly to my understanding of this problem; and to those who have contributed recipes: Annette Cowie, Emma Pilcher, Margie Turner, Cindy Ridden and Andra Somerville.

On the production side, special thanks to cartoonist Joanne Van Os; and to the team at Random House, especially editors Roberta Ivers and Lydia Papandrea, who were, as always, a pleasure to work with.

Finally, thanks again to my daughter Rebecca and son Arran for permitting their stories to be told and, of course, to my food technologist husband, Dr Howard Dengate for technical advice and, most of all, his constant support.

Contents

Introduction

I first noticed the asthma–food connection through my work with children's behaviour problems. When children did an elimination diet—free of additives and low in certain food chemicals—I asked families to follow the diet too, in order to support their children. Months later, parents would often mention that asthma in a family member had gone, and only recurred when they broke the diet. I was as surprised as they were.

As the years went by I continued to see remarkable improvements in asthmatics, even when the parents had previously said, 'but my child's asthma isn't related to food'.

In one such case a nine-year-old with severe asthma was referred for learning difficulties. His delighted mother phoned a year later after the annual checkup with a paediatrician:

> I didn't expect the diet to make any difference to his asthma because he's always had that. Now it's gone. He doesn't need his medication any more and he has normal lung function for the first time in his life.

I became increasingly puzzled. Could the answer really be as simple as food, I wondered, and if so, why hadn't researchers discovered this?

When I turned to the medical journals, I was gobsmacked. The link between food additives and asthma was recognised more than 25 years ago. Many experts discount the effects of additives because they expect a quick, obvious reaction. But most of the time, that's not the way it works, with either behaviour or asthma.

In children with difficult behaviour, continual exposure to food chemicals leads to irritability. If doing something they enjoy, these children will appear normal, but a request to do something they don't like—like 'it's time to do your homework'—can trigger an overreaction such as whining, oppositional defiance or spitting the dummy.

In children with asthma, continual exposure to food chemicals can lead to irritable airways. If kept away from triggers, these children will appear normal, but exposure to an environmental irritant—like a virus, pollen or dust mites—can trigger an overreaction of the airways, that is, an asthma attack.

Sulphite preservatives are to asthmatics what food colourings are to difficult children. They are not the only food chemicals which cause problems, but they are the additives most commonly associated with the condition and can sometimes trigger obvious asthma attacks.

Of all the preservatives in foods and drugs, sulphites (220–228) are probably the most frequently used. They have been responsible for many deaths, near deaths, and suffering. There are safer alternatives available for all foods except wine. If these harmful additives could be banned tomorrow, millions of asthmatics would improve without the need to change their diet.

However, sulphites aren't the only problem. Most asthmatics react to one or two food chemicals from the range of preservatives, colours, monosodium glutamate (MSG) and salicylates. Aspirin sensitivity has been recognised in asthmatics for a hundred years. Less well known is that salicylates in most fruits and some vegetables can also affect aspirin-sensitive asthmatics.

Because most foods today have high levels of additives, the relationship between additives and their effects are hidden. We can only see the effects of additives by trying one additive at a time while following a diet which avoids all other potentially harmful additives and food chemicals. I call this the FAILSAFE diet. Why FAILSAFE? Because it is Free of Additives and Includes Low Salicylates, Amines and Flavour Enhancers. The failsafe diet can help you to find out *which* foods are associated with your asthma, and *how* to avoid them. Please read on . . .

part
one

What Causes Asthma?

1 Asthma is increasing

Summary
- Asthma is increasing almost all over the world, and experts do not know why.
- Asthma is associated with the Western lifestyle, but air pollution, dust mites and smoking don't appear to be the main or even major factors.
- Experts are starting to say, could it be food?
- People who work with the failsafe diet see that the majority of asthmatics can improve if they change what they eat.
- Only a small percentage of asthmatics suffer attacks obviously triggered by foods.
- In some people, food chemicals can cause inflammation of the airways, called bronchial hyper-responsiveness (BHR). BHR can be symptom-free, but it is a strong risk factor for the development of asthma. People with BHR are more likely to react to environmental triggers like viruses, dust mites or pollen.
- Perhaps half of all adult asthmatics and two-thirds of children are affected by food additives. Processed food is a major contributing factor to world-wide asthma.
- Studies which claim only a small number of asthmatics are affected by foods have failed to use an effective elimination diet.

Asthma is increasing almost all over the world. In Australia, about two million people are affected by asthma. Approximately one in ten adults, one in seven teenagers, and one in four children are estimated to have asthma and the figures are still rising. In a 2001 survey, nearly half of all children surveyed had used a medicine for asthma in the previous year.

Until the 1950s asthma was rarely fatal. Not only is asthma increasing, it is increasing in severity. Over 950 Australians died of asthma in 1989, causing widespread alarm and prompting the establishment of the National Asthma Campaign (NAC), now the National Asthma Council, to reduce the death rate. The NAC was successful: the death rate dropped steadily to under 500 in the year 2000.

Despite this, Australia still has the second highest asthma death rate in the world. Our death rate is twice that of England.

You don't have to be a severe asthmatic to die of asthma. In Darwin, a man kissed his wife and young children goodnight before going to dinner with colleagues. His family would never see him alive again. After the meal he developed asthma and died. He wasn't even considered asthmatic. Many asthma death statistics hide similar tragedies.

A 15-year-old schoolgirl in Wagga Wagga suffered an asthma attack at school and died in the car on the way to hospital. She had not experienced an asthma attack since early childhood.

The NAC's strategy for reducing asthma deaths is to advise asthmatics to take preventive medication. Despite the NAC's reduction of the death rate, there has still been a dramatic increase in the prevalence of asthma. People in different regions think they are living in an 'asthma belt' with a particularly high rate of asthma. The reality is that there is no asthma belt: the incidence of asthma is increasing everywhere.

Researchers know that asthma is connected with the Western lifestyle, but they do not know why. They recognise that the key to the understanding and prevention of asthma lies with children. By comparing children in regions with different rates of asthma, they hope to understand the cause.

Not air pollution, dust mites, pollen or sprays

In developed countries, rates of asthma are the same in urban and rural areas. When city children in Melbourne were compared with country children in Victoria, the overall asthma rate was the same for city and country children, but there were variations between the country areas. Asthma rates were compared in five country regions representing known environmental factors:

- **air pollution**—La Trobe Valley, an industrial centre with coal mining and coal fired power plants, topped the asthma ratings. It was assumed to represent high air pollution until tests showed that air quality in La Trobe Valley at any given time was superior to air quality in Melbourne city, which had the third highest asthma.
- **agricultural sprays**—Mildura riverland area, representing agricultural sprays, had the second highest asthma.
- **garden pollens**—the highland region around Bright was selected for being low in dust mites and grass pollens, but with a range of garden pollens. It was fourth on the asthma scale.
- **dust mites**—with high dust mites and low pollen due to an onshore breeze, the coastal regions around Bairnsdale and Warrnambool had the second lowest asthma.
- **grass pollens**—the wheatbelt region around Horsham, representing high grass pollens, had the lowest asthma.

Researchers were dumbfounded. None of the sites thought to be highest in known environmental factors came out on top. La Trobe Valley wasn't highest in anything except asthma. Some researchers are starting to wonder if they are missing something. Could it be food?

The Saudi Arabian village study

The best place to study the increase in asthma is in a country where the change is still occurring—a society in transition—rather than one where it has become established.

Unlike developed countries, developing countries show a difference in asthma rates between city and rural children.

In Saudi Arabia, researchers compared village children eating a traditional diet based on rice, vegetables, lamb, chicken, dates, local fruits and milk with children in the oil boom city of Jeddah. City children ate more Western style processed foods from super-markets and fast food outlets. Asthma was two to three times more common in the city children than in the village children. Researchers concluded that eating Western style processed food *at least doubled and nearly tripled* the risk of asthma.

How to halve the rate of asthma

The reverse would seem to apply. If we want to reduce the prevalence of asthma by half to two thirds, all we have to do is avoid processed foods. Studies suggest that about 70 per cent of asthmatic children and 50 per cent of asthmatic adults react to at least one food additive. If asthmatics could live on a diet totally free of processed foods for a few weeks, would half of them improve? This is exactly what happened in a hospital study in Denmark.

The grey glop study

More than 40 chronic asthmatics (defined as at least one asthma attack per day of unknown origin) were admitted to hospital and divided into two groups. For two weeks, one group lived on an unflavoured additive-free elemental formula consisting only of essential nutrients. The other group ate disguised hospital food, diluted and blended to resemble the formula. All medications were additive free. The outcomes for the two groups were strikingly different.

In the hospital food group, only one patient improved, and three patients suffered life-threatening asthma attacks.

In the elemental formula group, *half improved significantly and none worsened*.

But don't worry. You don't have to live on grey glop to improve your asthma. The trick is to find an effective elimination diet.

Why hasn't my doctor told me about the elimination diet?

Most doctors are understandably reluctant to recommend dietary treatment of asthma. Medical journals are full of

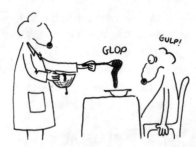

contradictions. For years, the issue of foods and asthma has been confused by the assumption that all reactions to foods are allergies. Reactions to food additives are *not* allergies. If they were allergies, they would be very easy to identify by simple tests. Instead, they are extremely difficult to identify (see p. 8).

In the 2002 update of their Asthma Management Handbook, the NAC acknowledges that asthma can be triggered by both allergies and intolerances, although noting that these are 'uncommon triggers' for asthma. While it is true that foods don't often *trigger* asthma attacks, what is not yet widely understood by most asthma experts is the hidden effect of food chemicals.

Most people expect that if food chemicals affect them, they will have an attack of asthma within 30 minutes. This is what happens with allergies. It also happens sometimes with unusually large doses of food additives or in exceptionally sensitive asthmatics. But for most asthmatics, foods do not trigger obvious attacks. What happens is much more subtle.

The effects of food chemicals are hidden

In some children, especially those with a family history of hayfever, asthma or eczema, food chemicals can cause irritable airways, called bronchial hyperresponsiveness (BHR). Adults can be affected too, especially women. A person can have BHR without any symptoms.

Individuals with BHR are more likely to react to environmental triggers such as viruses, dust mites or pollen. So when a mother says, 'But his asthma isn't related to foods, he only gets it when he has a cold', it is possible that certain food chemicals have made the child's airways more sensitive and the cold triggers an obvious attack. The underlying BHR and additives which contributed to it are not obvious. BHR is reduced when food chemicals to which the child is sensitive are avoided. The child can now have a cold without developing asthma.

FROM THE MEDICAL JOURNALS

'Exposure to [food chemicals] is sufficiently frequent to mask any relationship between ingestion and symptoms in susceptible people.'

Corder EH and Buckley CE, Aspirin, salicylate, sulfite and tartrazine induced bronchoconstriction. *J Clin Epidemiol* 1995;48(10):1269–75.

It is impossible to unravel the effects of food additives without using an elimination diet. *All* food chemicals likely to cause problems must be avoided for at least two weeks, preferably longer. This is to establish a low baseline. Otherwise, frequent consumption of food additives will produce a high level of background reactions in sensitive people. Against this, it is hard to distinguish the effects of any one particular additive. Once this low and stable baseline is established, any reaction can be clearly measured against the baseline. Most studies don't use a suitable elimination diet, which is why the effects of additives have been seriously underestimated for so long.

Light years ahead

In my experience, the best elimination diet in the world is the one I call failsafe, developed at the Royal Prince Alfred Hospital (RPAH) Allergy Clinic in Sydney during 20 years of research. A failsafe study of asthma and food chemicals from this clinic reminds me of *Dr Who*. From the outside it looks like an old-fashioned London phonebox. On the inside it is a sleek, hyper-advanced spaceship.

The study compared two methods of testing food chemicals on asthmatics: the traditional 'no-diet' method against the elimination diet method. For both methods, asthmatics took

Food allergy or food intolerance?

Food allergy is an immunological reaction to food proteins.
Food intolerance is a pharmacological reaction (like the side effects of a drug) to the chemicals in foods.

FAMILY HISTORY
Allergy: hayfever, eczema or asthma
Intolerance: migraine, irritable bowel symptoms, behaviour problems

WHO IS AFFECTED?
Allergies are most likely to affect babies and young children because of their underdeveloped immune system.
Food intolerance affects a much wider group. Children are vulnerable because dose for weight, they consume a higher dose of food chemicals than adults. Women of child–bearing age are vulnerable because of hormonal influence. Senior citizens are vulnerable because ageing livers and kidneys are slower to excrete chemicals from the body. Exposure to toxic chemicals, pharmaceutical drugs or illness such as gastrointestinal infection can increase sensitivity.

HOW COMMON?
Food allergies (not airborne allergies such as pollens) are considered to be relatively rare—affecting up to 8% of babies under 12 months, 3% of children under five, and less than 1% of adults.
Food intolerance is much more common, affecting babies (through breastmilk), children and adults. Some experts suggest 10% are affected, although, in theory, everyone will react if the dose is high enough, so you would expect more people to be affected as levels of additives rise.

WHICH FOODS?
People with **food allergies** typically react to one or two foods. Allergy is produced by a combination of susceptibility and exposure so allergens vary. In Japan, buckwheat, and in the Mediterranean countries, lentils, are common allergens. In Australia the most common foods are milk, soy, egg, peanut and fish. Allergies to the last two are more likely to last throughout life.
With **food intolerance**, food chemicals such as additives and some natural food chemicals are involved. These can be in many different foods. Asthmatics are most likely to be affected by

sulphite preservatives (220–228) in a wide range of foods and drugs including fruit–flavoured cordials and drinks, wine, bread, sausages, dried fruit and even some medications given to asthmatics (p. 57).

TIMING
Allergic reactions are quick. They usually occur within 30 minutes and are often easy to identify.
Food intolerance reactions can be delayed up to 48 hours or more. Identification of reactions can be difficult. When problem foods are consumed frequently symptoms can appear to be a chronic condition rather than a food reaction.

DOSE
Allergic reactions can be triggered by the tiniest amount of an allergen.
Intolerance reactions to food chemicals are dose–related. Some people are more sensitive than others.

SYMPTOMS
Allergic reactions can include itching, swelling, rash, spreading hives, vomiting, diarrhoea, breathing difficulties, collapse and death.
Intolerance reactions can be the same as above plus extra symptoms on pp. 73–4. Food chemicals may trigger an acute asthmatic attack, but more commonly, frequent exposure results in irritable airways. Food intolerance symptoms can come and go and change throughout life.

DIAGNOSIS
Food allergy: involves an immune response (called IgE) which can be identified by skin prick tests and confirmed by avoidance and challenge.
Food intolerance: there are no laboratory tests. The only way to identify provoking foods is through a comprehensive elimination diet and careful challenges.

capsules containing food chemicals or placebos. The challenges were double blind, which means that no-one involved in the tests knew what was in the capsules. Placebos can tell you if the study is measuring what it is meant to. If you don't get any placebo reactions, the study is excellent. A few placebo

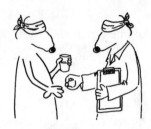

THE DOUBLE BLIND STUDY

reactions are okay because sometimes there are factors outside the researchers' control, but it is bad to get a lot of placebo reactions.

For the elimination diet method, the subjects followed the failsafe diet for four weeks then took the capsule challenges. The results were beautifully clear—11 reactions, no placebo reactions. The highest number of reactions were to the sulphite challenge, with eight (over 70 per cent) reacting, and one each to MSG, artificial colours and aspirin.

For the 'no-diet' method, as used in most studies, the subjects took the capsule challenges while eating a normal diet. The results were a mess—88 reactions including false negatives (no reaction where there should have been), false positives (reactions when there shouldn't have been) and lots of placebo reactions. Using this method, less than 20 per cent of subjects were shown to react to sulphites.

Expert opinions

This study is a perfect demonstration of why a suitable elimination diet must be used. The implications are huge: experts, including the US Food and Drug Administration, who say that only 5 per cent of asthmatics are sulphite sensitive, are mistaken.

There are two ways to follow a failsafe diet. One is to live in a Western society and restrict what you eat. The other is to live in a place where the local food is still failsafe. The few no-diet studies done in developing countries where residents can still eat a fairly failsafe diet may be more reliable than those in countries like the US where nearly all foods contain additives. When we look at studies that have been failsafe, either by accident or by design, they all tell the same story—sulphur-based preservatives affect a substantial number of asthmatics. In studies in both Papua New Guinea and South Africa, 40 per cent of asthmatics reacted to a sulphite challenge. In a failsafe study with children, mentioned above, the majority—nearly 70 per cent—reacted to sulphites.

It makes sense

With figures like these, all the other data starts to make sense. The difference between the Saudi children, the massive increase in asthma related to Western lifestyle and the big improvements attributed to the elimination diet, all fall into place.

How could doctors have been so mistaken for so long? It is very difficult to tease out the effects of foods. It took doctors 300 years to realise that scurvy was caused by a vitamin C deficiency. There is a joke that it takes 30 years for the results of research to reach doctors' surgeries. But this is no joke when you want answers for your own or your child's health now.

2 The asthma additive

Summary
- All over the world, researchers are working to discover the reason for the increase in asthma.
- The ISAAC (International Survey of Asthma and Allergies in Children) studies have reported the prevalence of asthma in 700,000 children in 56 countries.
- The challenge now is to explain the differences between countries. So far, studies looking at air pollution, dust mites, wealth, nutrition and other factors have not been able to do this.
- Processed food, and in particular variations in sulphite use, can explain the ISAAC findings.
- The regulation, monitoring and actual consumption of sulphites varies greatly between countries and can vary between regions within countries.
- It is possible to reduce sulphite levels in wine, and to ban sulphite use in other foods and medicines altogether. This could significantly reduce the prevalence of asthma.

Researchers all over the world are looking at the differences in asthma rates within countries and between countries. In the years 1994–95, a huge international project called ISAAC (International Survey of Asthma and Allergies in Children) looked at the prevalence of asthma in more than 700,000 city children in 56 countries. The results have puzzled researchers.

The ISAAC survey showed that the prevalence of asthma is increasing worldwide, that asthma is more prevalent in Western countries, that asthma prevalence increases in developing countries as they become more Westernised and that the highest asthma prevalence is in English-speaking countries. Spanish speaking countries also rate more highly than expected. A number of researchers have tried to explain the differences between countries by looking at air pollution, dust mites and nutrition.

Air pollution

If you ask any group of people what causes asthma, at least one person will say 'air pollution' but ISAAC surveys have shown that while air pollution contributes to bronchitis and pneumonia it is not a big factor in the development of asthma. Children from cities with exceptionally heavy air pollution in Russia, China and the former East Germany have surprisingly low rates of asthma. New Zealand has some of the cleanest air in the world and one of the highest rates of asthma. In the US, air quality has improved but the rates of asthma have not.

Dust mites

Although sensitisation to house dust mites is a risk factor for the development of asthma, it cannot explain increasing rates of asthma. A comparison of children in Hong Kong, Malaysia and southern China showed very different rates of asthma despite similar rates of dust mite allergens.

Smoking

While smoking or exposure to passive smoke can make asthmatics worse, smoking alone does not appear to contribute to the increase in asthma. In the comparison of the south-east

Asian regions above, the southern China region had the highest level of cigarette smoking and the lowest rate of asthma. In the US, the percentage of smokers has dropped over the last 30 years while asthma has increased steadily.

Nutrition

One study looked at the components of diet—except for additives—in every ISAAC listed country. Researchers found a strong association between the intake of starch, cereals and vegetables and low asthma rates. Diets of economically developed countries and urban areas of the developing world are relatively low in cereals and other starchy foods, and relatively

---

Prevalence of childhood asthma in children aged 13–14 according to the ISAAC questionnaire. The second figure is the wealth rating by gross national product.

Highest asthma— up to 30% of children	Medium asthma	Lowest asthma— down to 2% of children
1. UK 13	**19. Germany 4**	38. Oman 25
2. New Zealand 18	**20. France 6**	**39. Italy 10**
3. Australia 15	**21. Japan 1**	40. Pakistan 50
4. Irish Republic 17	22. Thailand 38	41. Latvia 39
5. Canada 8	**23. Sweden 3**	42. Poland 36
6. Peru 42	24. Hong Kong 14	43. Algeria 40
7. Costa Rica 37	25. Philippines 46	44. South Korea 22
8. Brazil 33	**26. Belgium 7**	45. Morocco 44
9. USA 2	**27. Austria 5**	46. Mexico 28
10. Paraguay 41	28. Iran n/a	47. Ethiopia 55
11. Uruguay 27	29. Argentina 24	48. India 53
12. Panama 34	30. Estonia 31	49. Taiwan 19
13. Kuwait 11	31. Nigeria 52	50. Russia 35
14. South Africa 32	32. Spain 16	51. China 49
15. Malta 21	33. Chile 29	52. Greece 23
16. Finland 12	**34. Singapore 9**	53. Georgia 48
17. Lebanon 26	35. Malaysia 30	54. Romania 43
18. Kenya 54	36. Portugal 20	55. Albania 51
	37. Uzbekistan 45	56. Indonesia 47

Top ten wealth ratings in bold

high in sugar, fat, protein of animal origin, salt, meat, dairy products and alcohol. The researchers could not work out why this should be related to asthma. They speculated about the protective effects of antioxidants like Vitamin E found in cereal, rice and vegetables but didn't mention the additives usually found in high sugar, high fat, high salt, processed foods and alcohol.

Since asthma is related to the Western lifestyle, you would expect the richest countries to have the highest rates of asthma. But this is not necessarily what researchers found. English-speaking Western countries had the highest asthma prevalences. Many Spanish and Portuguese speaking communities in Latin America had higher prevalences than in Spain and Portugal.

How did Italy become the only high wealth country in the low asthma column? What could put low wealth countries such as Peru and Paraguay in the asthmatic top ten along with high wealth Australia? And why doesn't the US, icon of the Western lifestyle, top the list?

These questions have researchers baffled. Clearly, factors other than wealth are involved. I suggest that those factors are food additives, especially—but not only—sulphites. Consumption of food additives varies from country to country in a way that can account for the variations.

Why is Italy in the low column?

Italians don't like food additives. Unlike people in English-speaking countries, Western Europeans, in general, prefer to avoid unnecessary additives. The European Union (EU) enforces strict rules and the Italians are particularly additive-conscious. After the introduction of food colourings and preservatives in the '70s, a consumer campaign in Italy led to public outcry. The use of food additives was reduced. Labels boasting *senza coloranti, senza additivi* (without colours, without additives) are common on packaged foods. Today, about 95 per cent of a confectionery display in a big Italian supermarket will typically be additive free, compared to less than 5 per cent in Australian, English or American supermarkets.

According to an Italian survey, the foods most likely to contribute sulphites in the Italian diet are wine for adults and dried fruit for children. Although the EU permits the use of sulphites in processed meat such as sausages, researchers found that, in general, Italians do not use sulphites in meat and meat products.

Italy's concern about food additives may be paying off. In 2001, a survey of Rome schoolchildren announced that the dramatic increase in childhood asthma—a three-fold increase over two decades from 1974—appears to have come to an end. This is in striking contrast to most other ISAAC countries whose asthma rates are still increasing.

What about Peru and Paraguay?

Peru and Paraguay are the only low wealth countries to make it into the asthmatic top ten, just behind Australia, leaving most researchers shaking their heads in bewilderment. But there is a connection: all of those countries eat meat as a staple, use sulphites to preserve meat, and show poor compliance with food regulations.

Australia and Paraguay were the first countries in the world to use sulphites as meat preservatives, back in colonial days when they shipped meat back to Britain and Spain. In Australia today, sulphites are permitted in sausages, and limits can be exceeded. Although sulphites are not permitted in fresh minced meat, this regulation too is sometimes disregarded.

Similarly, analyses of sausages and burgers in Spain found excessive use of sulphites. Most samples were over the limit and some were well over, up to *16 times the legal amount* of sulphites. Spain's use of sulphites is now in line with EU regulations, but it is reasonable to assume that her former colonies are not. Since fresh meat is so expensive, the most popular form of meat, in Peru at least, is the sulphite-preserved *chorizo* or spicy Spanish sausage.

From the asthma point of view, it doesn't matter whether your intake of sulphites comes entirely from one source— for example, a serve of sausages containing high levels of sulphites—or from many different processed foods containing small levels of sulphites. Unlike other English-speaking and Spanish-speaking countries, the US has a total ban on the use of sulphites in meat. However, there are other ways of getting sulphites into consumers.

Why doesn't the US top the table?

You would expect the country with the most Western lifestyle in the world to have by far the highest asthma rate. Instead, the US comes ninth, between Peru and Paraguay. How can this be? I suggest that the US, through using outrageously high amounts of sulphites, was the first country to find out just exactly how dangerous these additives are.

In the 1980s in America there were at least 27 publicised asthma deaths related to sulphites, and over a thousand reports of serious reactions. Most were linked with excessive use of sulphites sprayed on salads to keep them looking fresh.

Alarmed by these reactions, a non-profit consumer organisation called Center for Science in the Public Interest (CSPI) campaigned for a total ban on the use of sulphites as food additives. After four years, the Food and Drug Administration (FDA) compromised by prohibiting the use of sulphites on fruits—except grapes—and on vegetables that are sold raw or likely to be eaten raw.

I believe this single change in regulations has saved many lives and avoided many asthma attacks, and has probably saved US children from topping the list. The FDA also tried to stop the use of sulphites on fresh potatoes to be cooked and served as unlabelled French fries, but was defeated after a long court battle with the potato industry.

Although these regulations have discouraged some large amounts of sulphites, there are low levels of sulphites in virtually all processed food. After studying nearly 2500 American asthmatics at the Allergy-Immunology Clinic of Duke University Medical Center, researchers expressed their concern about 'the prevalence and abundance of unlabeled sulphites' in US foods.

The most common source of sulphites in processed foods is refined corn products, made from corn which has been soaked in a sulphite solution. This includes corn syrup, which is the top-selling sweetener in the US, with per person consumption quadrupling over the last thirty years. Sugar is no safer, as in the US it is usually made from sulphite-soaked sugar beets, rather than from sugar cane. Another common sweetener, grape juice concentrate, is also a source of sulphites as grapes are the one raw fruit on which sulphites are still permitted. Although the amounts of sulphites are small, these ingredients are in many products and it all adds up.

Alternatives 'possible'

The Italian survey concluded that it may be possible to find alternatives to sulphites for all foods except wine. Residues in wine have been reduced due to improved technology, but even with the reduced sulphite rates of 75 mg/L (milligrams per litre) now found in France, French researchers noted that adults could exceed the acceptable daily intake—which is absolutely no guarantee of safety for an asthmatic—by drinking four small glasses of wine a day.

The Australian maximum permitted level for wine is 250 mg/L, although it is possible to get quality white wines with a range of 90–120 mg/L and reds with a range of 50–70 mg/L. An asthmatic teenager who had never heard of sulphites was pleased to know there was an explanation for his observation, 'I get asthma 15 minutes after drinking cask wine, but I don't have a problem with my dad's expensive bottled stuff'.

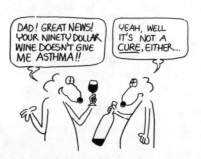

The use of sulphites and other additives in processed foods is a more plausible explanation for the increase and variation in asthma worldwide than any other proposal so far. It would be interesting to compare actual consumption of sulphites and other additives in all 56 ISAAC countries. Perhaps ISAAC researchers will examine it soon. As we have seen, there is a big difference between how many sulphites a country allows and what actually reaches the consumer. Sulphites can be reduced by cooking or time standing on the shelf. Manufacturers will sometimes compensate for this by adding well over the legal limit and assuming the level will reduce by purchase date. The only way to determine the actual consumption of additives is to carry out analyses of foods as in the Italian survey mentioned before.

But there's no need to wait for ISAAC researchers to discover the effects of sulphites. You could be asthma-free in a few weeks. All you have to do is find out which food chemicals affect your asthma and learn to avoid them.

3 Sulphites up close and personal

Summary

- Sulphite preservatives (220–228) can cause fatal reactions in large doses or in extra sensitive people.
- Obvious reactions to sulphites are only the tip of the iceberg.
- Sulphites are the most common—but not the only—additives which can affect asthmatics.
- Sulphites are used in most processed foods and many drugs.

Karen's story is a classic sulphite reaction. She and her boyfriend ate burgers and fries at a fast food outlet. 'About 10 minutes after we finished eating, my throat began to itch,' Karen recalls. 'I grabbed my inhaler but I could feel my throat constricting. I couldn't breathe and started to panic. When I passed out, my boyfriend flagged down a passing police car. The officer radioed for an ambulance, and I was rushed to the hospital. I was revived with a massive dose of epinephrine.'

The trigger in this case was the fries. Potatoes are often soaked in a sulphite solution after peeling. Karen, 37, had reacted to sulphites before and knew to avoid wine, shrimps, and 'other foods that contain sulphites'. But she didn't know enough to avoid fries, and it nearly killed her.

Most reactions aren't obvious

In a survey of more than 80 asthmatic adults in Melbourne, the foods most commonly reported as causing asthma were red wine, pickled onions and gherkins, fruit cake (with dried fruit), and sausages/frankfurters. These all contain significant quantities of sulphites (more details on p. 188) but only a few asthmatics experience dramatic reactions like Karen. Most do not realise they are affected.

In a study of thousands of American asthmatics, researchers at Duke University Medical Center identified two groups of sulphite sensitive asthmatics: those who know they react to sulphites and those who don't. Asthmatics in the second—much larger—group have subclinical reactions, that is, no obvious symptoms. The researchers concluded that *people who are severely sensitive to sulphites may be better off in the long term because they notice reactions and will avoid exposure*. The majority, those who are unaware of the effects of sulphites, may develop chronically inflamed lungs over the long term and are at greater risk of lung function impairment.

This is what happened to Liz. Now 41, she has suffered from asthma most of her life. For over 30 years she took 'just about every drug' and spent many weeks in hospital, always ending up on cortisone, but she didn't realise she was affected by sulphites.

> Sometimes I would eat or drink something and then feel wheezy and tight in the chest, but another time the same food would be okay. I could never pinpoint it exactly. No-one in the medical profession ever suggested to me, 'it could be what you are eating'.
>
> One day I had a very bad asthma attack after eating salami and French onion dip. Within five minutes the top of my mouth became tingly, I was sitting on the toilet and my throat and lips had swollen so much that I couldn't breathe. By the time I arrived in hospital I had lost control of my bowels (very embarrassing) and my peak flow [lung function] was non-existent. I ended up having a week of skin prick tests and swallowing capsules in hospital and that is how I found out that I reacted to metabisulphite.
>
> I cut out all foods containing metabisulphite, including sausages, all processed deli meat, cordials, jams, shop produced fruit salad, anything pickled with vinegar, shop bought hot chips, dried foods like apricots and anything that isn't natural. Occasionally I come across food that I didn't realise had metabisulphite in it, like frozen apple pies and filled chocolates.
>
> Having asthma is a normal part of my life, and now I know one of the main triggers it makes a huge difference. Since I stopped eating food with metabisulphite in it five years ago I haven't had an asthma attack. I still take my medication, but I am healthy and happy.

Very few studies have looked at the effects of sulphites on children. This seems odd when you consider that children have more asthma than adults, and that children are more vulnerable to the effects of food additives.

In South Africa, a study conducted by the University of Cape Town found that over 40 per cent of asthmatic children reacted to a challenge of apple juice preserved with sulphur dioxide.

The Sydney Children's Hospital study

At the Children's Hospital in Sydney, a study using a much more comprehensive elimination diet than usual showed just how many asthmatic children can be affected by sulphites. All 29 children were chosen for their chronic moderate-to-severe asthma rather than dietary history. All were receiving continuous preventer and reliever medication and most of them had never noticed a reaction to foods. According to the US Food and Drug Administration (FDA) estimates, only *5 per cent* of the children would be expected to react to metabisulphite challenge. Instead, a clear majority, nearly *70 per cent* (19 children) reacted to metabisulphite within 30 minutes of the challenge. Only seven of the reactors had previously noticed that they reacted to foods. Pickled onions and a particular brand of orange juice were the foods most commonly identified. Both contain metabisulphite.

Delayed reactions

Two of the children had no reaction during the laboratory tests, however both had reactions that same night. They were assumed to be delayed reactors, but were not counted in the study. They would have brought the count to *72 per cent* responding.

The RPAH Allergy Clinic study mentioned in Chapter 1 also contained a delayed reactor. The woman had previously reported that if she drank wine with dinner she would have asthma the next day. At a rough estimate based on both studies, 10 per cent of reactions were delayed. People always tend to blame the food last eaten, so delayed reactions can be confusing.

When six-year-old Robert did the elimination diet for stomach aches, his asthma cleared up as well. One evening several months later he ate off-diet sausages which led to irritable bowel symptoms that night. After breakfast the next morning Robert had asthma for the first time since starting the diet. His mother's first response was, 'it can't be anything he ate, he had the same breakfast as he always does.' Sausages are a common source of

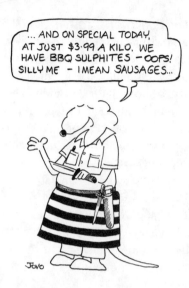

... AND ON SPECIAL TODAY,
AT JUST $3·99 A KILO, WE
HAVE BBQ SULPHITES −OOPS!
SILLY ME − I MEAN SAUSAGES...

sulphites in the diets of young children. Robert's mother had
never noticed an asthmatic reaction to any food. The elimination
diet enabled her to identify the effect of sulphites on Robert's
asthma.

A sulphite-free diet

Compared to the families I have worked with, the sulphite
reactors in the Children's Hospital study had a disappointing
response to diet. They were asked to follow a sulphite-free diet
for three months. Nearly half of them reported that they felt
better, but only one-fifth achieved normal lung function. Since
colours, MSG and dairy foods were excluded from the original
two-week diet, but not tested by challenge, there is a good
chance that at least some of the children in this study were
reacting to other additives or foods in their diets. Or their
sulphite-free diets may not have been as low in sulphites as
expected. The researchers commented that the sulphite-free diet
'did not involve radical changes in food consumption', and
sulphite-free alternatives could be 'substituted with ease'.
I don't agree, and nor does Rick Williams, a sulphite-sensitive
computer expert from California who runs the NoSulfites

website. 'In modern America,' he says, 'sulphites are every-where and avoiding them is a very complicated task.'

Although regulations are becoming stricter, in Australia sulphites do not have to be declared if the sulphite content of the product is: less than 10 ppm (parts per million); in an ingredient which is less than 5 per cent of the total product; sold unpackaged, like sausages and prawns, or in takeaways and in restaurant food—or if the manufacturer is prepared to take the very small risk of being caught.

The easiest way to avoid sulphites is to avoid *all* additives—and processed foods—like the asthmatic adults in a Swiss study. Nearly 45 per cent reacted to sulphites and 20 per cent to other additives. A completely additive-free diet resulted in marked improvement within five days and was still effective at follow up 14 months later.

This is what happened, by accident, to my family. When my daughter was two, we moved to Wagga Wagga, a wheatbelt town in New South Wales. Every spring, when thunderstorms bearing high pollen counts sweep across the plains, scores of asthmatics literally run into hospital emergency rooms. My daughter Rebecca, husband Howard and I were diagnosed with asthma within two years of our arrival, and our baby, Arran, was diagnosed later.

Rebecca's asthma started with a persistent night cough and progressed to exercise-induced asthma. Since sports such as bushwalking and skiing were a big part of our life, we had to carry a puffer at all times and Rebecca's asthma disrupted our lives.

After the move to Wagga Wagga, our diet changed from the wholefood, mostly vegetarian diet we had eaten in New Zealand. We started eating more processed foods and takeaways but, like most asthmatics, we never noticed any effect of food on our asthma. A leaflet from our doctor assured us that diet played no part in asthma.

Rebecca's asthma was obviously triggered by exercise, Howard's by pollens, and mine by pollens, cigarette smoke and hairspray. Arran just seemed like a wheezy baby.

At about the same time, Howard's mother suggested the

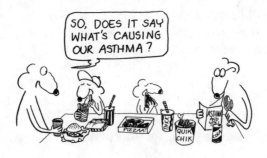

Pritikin diet to prevent the heart disease which was a problem in their family. After living with asthma for a year, we started the Pritikin diet. Avoiding fats, sugars and most processed foods also meant no additives. During our final year in Wagga Wagga, we enjoyed the health benefits of our new diet: I lost 15 kg; Howard and I achieved low cholesterol levels; and Rebecca's behaviour improved, although it would be years before we found the answer to that puzzle. Almost as an afterthought, as in so many of the families I see, we gradually realised that asthma was no longer a problem.

A sulphite challenge

At the end of the year, we spent an interesting six weeks driving across Australia to a new job in tropical Darwin. In one outback town we stopped for 'pure' fruit icecreams. Within minutes we were all coughing and gasping. Sulphites are used to preserve fruit pulp. We had just experienced our first very obvious sulphite reaction.

Our story is typical of the majority of asthmatics. We had been unaware of our sulphite sensitivity. When we went additive-free, our asthma disappeared. It took a large dose of sulphites while on an elimination diet to demonstrate a reaction. Previously, frequent small amounts of sulphites had provoked an asthmatic condition which seemed to be triggered by environmental factors.

In the 14 years since, we have stuck to our additive-free and later failsafe diet. Rebecca and I have had no asthma at all. Howard has experienced 'in-flight coughing' a few times after eating fruit salad on planes. Arran has experienced a few mild asthmatic episodes after walking past heaps of sulphur on a wharf, and on one occasion while showering in sulphurous bore water in central Queensland.

FROM THE MEDICAL JOURNALS

In Australia, a 67–year–old asthmatic nearly died after eating tinned crabmeat salad with vinegar based dressing. Two weeks after recovery she was readmitted to hospital for elimination and food challenges. There was no reaction to tinned crabmeat or any food additive except sodium metabisulphite which is present in vinegar. Except for one mistake, on a strict sulphite–free diet, no further attacks occurred.

Summarised from Baker GJ and others, Bronchospasm induced by metabisulphite–containing foods and drugs, *Med J Aust* 1981;2(11):614–17.

In Canada, a 27–year–old worker with no previous history of asthma developed occupational asthma after just three to four weeks in a new job. His work involved cleaning potatoes with water and sprinkling them with dried metabisulphite powder.

Summarised from Malo JL and others, Occupational asthma caused by dry metabisulphite, *Thorax* 1995;50(5):585–6.

Asthma currently costs the Australian community about $700 million a year. We know that sulphites affect asthmatics. We know that alternatives can be found for sulphites in all foods except wine, and that those in wine can be minimised.

I agree with American scientists from the Center for Science in the Public Interest. Sulphites as food additives should be banned. But the food industry will never consent. Instead, they will argue forever about just how many asthmatics are affected. As the FDA found with potatoes, regulators don't seem strong enough to regulate the food industry.

It is up to us consumers. Together we have the power. The answer is simple. *Refuse to buy*. If enough consumers avoid products preserved with sulphites, there will be a mad scramble for change by the food industry. And it might just save your life.

4 Colour me asthmatic

Summary

- Artificial food colours have been associated with asthma for more than 40 years.
- Although tartrazine (102, yellow #5) is the worst, all artificial colours and several natural colours can cause problems.
- Effects of additives are related to dose. The more you eat, the more likely you are to be affected.
- Long before there is an obvious reaction, additives can cause irritable airways which makes the asthmatic more susceptible to other triggers.
- Most asthmatics are unaware of the effects of additives until they do an elimination diet.
- Tartrazine and other additives can pass through breastmilk to affect babies. They can also be absorbed through the skin from lotions, toiletries and enemas.
- The use of colours in processed foods is increasing.
- Artificial colours should be banned in foods consumed by children as they can do harm and serve no necessary function.

Ryan Perry was introduced to tartrazine yellow colour in a flavoured milk at the age of 19 months. Within minutes he had an asthma attack so severe that teams of doctors from two hospitals had to work for hours to save his life. Eventually he came around but, according to his mother, 'it was very dicey'.

So far, 36 people have notified the US Food and Drug Administration of similar reactions to tartrazine (102, yellow #5). People with severe reactions like Ryan's are the tip of the iceberg. Extreme reactions in a few are an indication of milder reactions in many. There are asthmatics eating tartrazine every day who have never realised its effect on them.

In Australia, a man used asthma medication for 40 years. It took recognition of his daughter's sensitivity to tartrazine, plus an asthma attack triggered by his favourite dessert, for him to realise that his lifelong asthma was related to tartrazine.

In the beginning

The first report of colour-related asthma—six cases in children—was published in 1958. Nine years later a case of severe, chronic asthma was blamed on tartrazine in medications and yellow-coated vitamin tablets. These were followed by increasing reports of reactions, including asthma, to food colours and other additives. At this time, the use of food additives was just starting to become widespread in the US.

Processed food as we know it began in the US after World War I. No longer supplying the military with jams, jellies and preserves, the food industry pursued a new goal: selling large quantities of cheap food. The development of a refined pectin made it possible to make jelly using sugar and water alone. Artificial colours and flavours took care of the rest. Real foods like fruit were no longer necessary.

It is easier to notice effects when food additives are eaten infrequently. In 1955, production of food colours amounted to 12 mg per person per day, only a quarter of today's rate. This explains why there are more reports of food additive reactions in medical journals in the '60s and '70s, when doctors had a better chance to see what was happening.

FROM THE MEDICAL JOURNALS

'Tests for sensitivity to . . . food additives should be conducted as a routine measure for asthmatics.'

Stenius BS and Lemola M, Hypersensitivity to acetylsalicylic acid (ASA) and tartrazine in patients with asthma, *Clin Allergy* 1976;6(2):199–209.

When food additives are eaten frequently, the effects are hidden. Asthmatics are most likely to experience irritable airways which appears to be unrelated to food. As doses increase, so do the number of people with asthma.

The food industry has spent huge amounts of money on convincing people that artificial colours are harmless. It has worked. The FDA denies that artificial food colours cause any problems other than hives. Their pamphlet on food colours was co-sponsored with an industry trade association and described as 'misleading' by the Center for Science in the Public Interest, a group of scientists who scrupulously avoid industry involvement.

Food colours are not harmless

Asthma is not the main reaction to food colours, but it does happen. In an English study at the University of Surrey, all of a group of 23 hyperactive children reacted within two hours to a tartrazine yellow challenge with restlessness (18), aggression (16), poor coordination (12), asthma/eczema (8), violence (4) or poor speech (2).

The curry connection

Over the last 20 years, curries have become England's most popular dish. In 1999, health officials investigated a number of complaints about asthma and other 'allergies' from patrons in West Midlands curry restaurants.

They found that more than half the dishes surveyed contained excessive use of artificial colours. Tartrazine (102), sunset yellow (110) and ponceau red (124) were used in many dishes. There is no regulation covering the use of artificial colours in meat and rice dishes, but some curries contained up to 16 times the amount of colour recommended in similar sauces. As manager of a chain of seven colour-free curry houses, Mohammed Aslam says that many British curry fans do not realise how much colouring is being used. 'That's how they have been introduced to the food and they think that's how things are supposed to look. Indian cooking doesn't need artificial colouring because you can create the colours you want with spices.'

A sudden big increase in the use of additives is the best way to notice a reaction, which is what happened in the curry houses. Usually, the increase is gradual and children are most at risk. How many children exceed recommended doses through eating a combination of highly coloured foods? We have no idea. The actual consumption of food additives is rarely monitored.

Even breastfed babies are at risk from food additives because artificial colours and other food chemicals can pass through breastmilk. Although the usual reactions are irritability, restlessness, difficulty settling to sleep, frequent waking, skin rashes or frothy stools, asthma is possible.

Baby Joe's asthmatic cough started on day three, when his mother's milk came in. He also screamed constantly. His family now realises that food chemicals were the problem.

A GP put him on antibiotics at four months, thinking his screaming might be an infection of some sort. That's when the breathing problems and wheezing started. He was on

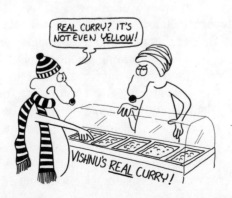

the nebuliser at least twice a day with corticosteroids, ipra-
troprium and salbutamol and oral steroids thrown in here
and there when he got really bad. He had all the tests for
causes—dust mites etc—which proved negative. Then he
started solids at five months and only got worse. When he
was two-and-a-half we started him on the elimination diet.
His asthma disappeared in the second week.

Challenges showed that Joe reacted to sulphites, benzoates,
nitrates and colours. One musk stick (azorubine 122 and erythrosine 127) started him coughing and wheezing within three
minutes. Annatto natural yellow colour (160b) took a little
longer. Tartrazine turned out to be the worst of all. Through
experience, his family learned that he gets asthma from
coloured antibiotics and coloured toothpaste. Additives can also
be absorbed through the skin. Joe gets asthma from playdough
made with food colours, coloured shampoo and coloured 'soap
on tap'.

Colours in medication

Most people forget about additives in medication. It isn't just
children who are affected. Now in her seventies, Ellie suffered
from asthma for 35 years, with numerous life-threatening
attacks and three episodes in intensive care. Her daughter
recalls, 'Mum was always in hospital and sometimes they
couldn't tell us whether she would last the night.' Ten years ago,
Ellie discovered the elimination diet for herself. She realised
that the drugs her doctor gave her in hospital contained an artificial red colour which made her asthma worse.

Since doing the elimination diet, Ellie has avoided acute
attacks except for a few mistakes including sulphited chips from
a fish and chip shop and the natural MSG in a Vegemite
sandwich. She is not able to give up corticosteroids because
'when you've had asthma as long as I have, you can't undo the
lung damage'.

Food colours can be found in a wide range of processed
foods. In the US, a desperate mother discovered that both her
breastfed baby's sleep patterns and her toddler's behaviour

improved when she avoided tartrazine. She had been eating tartrazine colour herself and feeding it to her two-year-old in potato, bread, yoghurt, canned soup, margarine, cough syrup, cakes, donuts, muffins, icecream, cookies, crackers, drink mixes, lemonade, pudding mix, boxed meals, rice and pasta dishes, cheesecake, butterscotch candy, jelly and chips.

Artificial food colours are unnecessary and potentially harmful. At the end of the twentieth century, the Center for Science in the Public Interest conducted a massive quarter century review of the effects of foods on behaviour. This is the same unbiased group of scientists who alerted the FDA to the dangers of sulphites.

Their conclusions were unequivocal. Some foods can affect some children's behaviour very badly indeed. The government, health professionals and others who are supposedly concerned for the welfare of children should take diet seriously. Fast food chains, food manufacturers, schools and paediatric hospitals should minimise the use of food additives which can cause behavioural problems. The FDA should 'consider banning the use of synthetic dyes in foods widely consumed by children *because dyes adversely affect some children and do not offer any essential benefits*'. Asthmatic kids would benefit from these recommendations too.

Food colours most likely to affect asthmatics

Artificial colours are called coal tar dyes because they were originally made from coal tar. Some coal tar dyes are also described as azo—a Greek word meaning 'without life'—because of their particular chemical structure. Azo dyes were the first to be recognised as harmful and a number were banned for carcinogenicity during the twentieth century. But products which claim to contain 'no azo dyes' may contain other harmful colours.

Natural colours are made from plant, animal or mineral extracts, but being natural is no guarantee of safety. Annatto extract is made from the seed coat of the tropical Annatto tree. In one study of 60 patients with urticaria (hives), more than twice as many reacted to annatto (26 per cent) than to tartrazine

(11 per cent). The worst artificial colour was sunset yellow, followed by three artificial reds. Natural red colour cochineal (carmine) is made from the body of a scale insect. It can cause severe allergic reactions including asthma and anaphylaxis.

AVOID THESE COLOURS

Coal tar dyes

102 *azo*	tartrazine *yellow*	
104	quinoline yellow	
110 *azo*	sunset yellow	
122 *azo*	carmoisine (azorubine) *red*	
123 *azo*	amaranth *red*	
124 *azo*	ponceau *red*	
127	erythrosine *red*	
132	indigotine *blue*	
133	brilliant blue	
142	food green	
151 *azo*	brilliant black	
155 *azo*	chocolate brown	

Synthetic but not a coal tar dye

129	allura red

Natural

160b	annatto *yellow* (beta–carotene 160a is safe)
120	cochineal *red* (allergic not intolerance reactions)

Natural colours cost more because the materials for them have to be grown on a farm instead of made in a laboratory. In the US, so much colour is used in manufactured foods that the food industry considers 'it is not currently reasonable to expect that the color could all be supplied from natural sources'. In Westernised countries, food colours have gone way beyond additives in confectionery and junk food. They are now even added to chicken feed to enhance the yellow colour of eggs and chicken skin, and to fish feed to enhance the colour of farmed salmon. Yet there are still enlightened countries like Italy or developing countries where colours are never added to foods.

How many react?

How many asthmatics react to artificial colours? We don't know. Studies suggest from zero to 30 per cent. We know that studies without elimination diets are likely to underestimate the prevalence. There is also confusion about dose.

As we saw in the English curry houses, if you increase the dose, noticeably more asthmatics will react. In the RPAH study mentioned in Chapter 1, approximately 70 per cent of patients reacted to sulphites and only 10 per cent to colours. While this suggests that sulphites are more commonly associated with asthma, the size of the colour challenge dose was a smallish 60 mg.

Researchers in the area of children's behaviour originally used low doses of 26 mg of colours per day. A study using 150 mg of colours showed many more children reacted. This higher dose was considered a realistic estimate of what some children ate in a day in 1976. Since then the production of food colours has increased by nearly 50 per cent. A realistic estimate of daily intake now, nearly 30 years later, would be much higher.

Food colours around the world

In developing countries like Nepal, you will never encounter a food colour outside major cities and tourist routes.

In Europe, artificial food colours are not used in local foods. They appear only in processed foods from large and multinational food manufacturers. Even then, many fewer harmful additives are used. The safe yellow colour beta-carotene (160a) is used widely instead of annatto or artificial colours. For example, in Australia, a popular orange coloured soft drink is coloured with sunset yellow. In European countries the same brand is coloured with either orange juice or beta-carotene (160a). In Italy, all those delicious gelati icecreams are coloured with real fruit.

In Britain, there is a greater awareness of the harmful effects of food colours than in Australia. Supermarket giant Sainsburys has a policy of reducing unnecessary additives, and carry bags from Iceland supermarkets boast: *'We have banned artificial colours and flavours.'*

In Australia, the use of artificial colours is increasing although it is not yet as extensive as in the US. Foods which contained no colours or natural colours a few years ago now contain artificial colours. This includes some breakfast cereals and many chocolate products.

The use of natural colour annatto (160b) is so widespread in Australia it is difficult to avoid, even in relatively healthy foods. Most yoghurts and light natural icecreams contain this colour as well as some healthy breakfast cereals. Although annatto is permitted in butter it is not used here yet, unlike the US. Australian regulators say it is too difficult and expensive to use beta-carotene (160a) which is a safe alternative to annatto, although betacarotene is used extensively throughout Europe.

It is in the US where food companies have really upped the ante and this is spreading to Australia. Drinks that turn your tongue green are big business and in one giant mystery promotion, pink, orange or teal coloured ketchup was camouflaged in squirt bottles so consumers couldn't tell which colour they were buying.

History shows that affluence often leads to decadence. While the most powerful nation in the world plays games with bizarrely coloured food, asthmatics are often the victims.

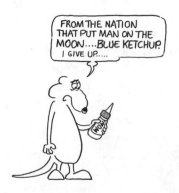

5 More preservatives

Summary
- Altogether 50 food additives have been identified as most likely to cause intolerance reactions.
- Other than sulphites, benzoates are the best known—but not the only—preservatives associated with asthma.
- Sensitivity to more than one food additive makes the task of identifying problem chemicals much more difficult.

A woman in her thirties was drinking two to three litres of cola a day. In an effort to lose weight, she changed to diet cola for three months. She had her first breathless attack in the middle of the night and thought she was dying. It took two more episodes and a diagnosis of asthma before she made the connection with the diet cola. Now I'm not advocating the overuse of cola, but she reverted to the regular cola and has had no further episodes.

What's in diet cola that isn't in regular cola? Aspartame artificial sweetener (951) and preservative sodium benzoate (211). While the safety of aspartame is questionable, benzoate preservative is most likely to be the culprit. It was first associated with asthma about 30 years ago.

Benzoates
Benzoates are commonly used in drinks. Like the incidence of asthma, the consumption of soft drinks has doubled in the last two decades. As well as containing artificial colours, most soft drinks—even natural mineral water with 5 per cent fruit juice—are preserved with sodium benzoate. So are the cordials and fruit drinks consumed instead of water by numerous children. For example, the additives in a typical lime-flavoured cordial drink—even with a percentage of real fruit—gives you four chances to aggravate your asthma with preservatives sodium benzoate (211) and sodium metabisulphite (223) along with colours 102 (tartrazine) and 133 (brilliant blue).

In 1996, a medical journal reported the case of an asthmatic girl treated with continuous medication from the age of one for six years. At that time, she experienced more frequent and severe attacks despite increased medication. Additive challenges showed sensitivity to benzoates. Avoidance of benzoates in drinks and medication resulted in complete disappearance of her asthmatic symptoms, and normal lung function.

Altogether, 50 additives (p. 231) have been associated with adverse reactions. These include colours, preservatives, antioxidants used to preserve oils, and flavour enhancers.

**PRESERVATIVES MOST LIKELY TO CAUSE
ADVERSE REACTIONS**

200–203	sorbates (*in dairy foods, fruit drinks and products*)
210–213	benzoates (*in juices, soft drinks, medications*)
220–228	sulphites (*wide range of foods and medications*)
280–283	propionates (*in breads, cheese, fruit and vegetable products*)
249–252	nitrates, nitrites (*in processed meats*)

Antioxidants (*in oils, margarines, fried foods and snack foods, not always listed*)

310–312	Gallates
319–321	TBHQ, BHA, BHT

Antioxidants

Most antioxidants such as Vitamin C and Vitamin E (additives 300–309) are healthy and are thought to protect us against cancer but antioxidants in the range 310–312 (gallates) and 319–321 (TBHQ, BHA and BHT) can affect asthmatics. They are used to stop fats and oils from going rancid. These additives are widespread and not always listed on the label, thanks to a five per cent labelling loophole (see page 203). Effects are cumulative and tiny amounts can build up. New Zealanders are particularly at risk. Antioxidants 319 and 320 have been so widely accepted in New Zealand that most vegetable oils and products containing vegetable oil—including bread—contain at least one of these potentially harmful additives.

BHT is widely used in the US, but permitted only in walnut and pecan kernels, cereal packets and polyethylene film food

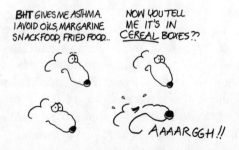

wrap in Australia and New Zealand. When used in packaging, it migrates into food.

A REACTION TO BHT

About a month after going on the diet, I ate some puffed rice breakfast cereal without looking at the label on the packet. I just assumed that cereals were OK. Within 30 minutes, I was wheezing, had hives, was itching and my eyes swelled.

I thought, this certainly couldn't be the cereal, but it was the only thing that I had consumed different that day. When I looked at the label on the box, it said that the packaging had BHT in it. I figured that the BHT from the packaging was enough to get into the cereal and give me that reaction.

Just to be certain that it wasn't the malt in the cereal that I was reacting to, I went to the health food store and bought some plain puffed rice with just rice and sugar, no preservatives, etc . . . and I didn't react. From that moment on, I tried to make sure that I didn't ingest BHT or BHA.—*Reader, from the US.*

Nitrates and nitrites (249–252)

Nitrates and nitrites are used as preservatives and colourants in processed meats like bacon, ham and devon. Baby Joe, in the last chapter, reacted to these preservatives. They can affect asthmatics very badly indeed. There is a report of nitrate-induced anaphylaxis on p. 144.

Propionates (280–283)

The use of calcium propionate (282) as a preservative in bread became widespread in Australia in the early 1990s. It is almost universal in the US, increasing in the UK but rarely used in Europe.

Since most people in Australia eat bread every day, children can be affected all of their lives without anyone realising. Babies can be affected through breastmilk. Effects usually build up slowly. Propionates are one of the additives least associated with asthma, but it can happen.

My study about effects of the bread preservative on children's behaviour was published in a medical journal in 2002. Since then

I have been contacted by people all over Australia telling me how much they improved after switching to preservative-free bread. One delighted mother phoned after six weeks. As well as other improvements, she described how the three asthmatics in the family, herself and two children, had been asthma-free for the last three weeks, 'and that's a *really* long time for us.'

> 'You need an observant patient and a physician with the mind of Sherlock Holmes to work out the effects of food additives.'

So many additives

Food additives are now eaten so frequently that a relationship between consumption and symptoms is no longer obvious. Don't forget, additives can be in both foods and medications.

In a remote town, seven-year-old Emily developed a night cough following a flu. While she was at home from school recovering, her mother gave her a packet of snack food as a treat, 'the first time she's ever had it'. Emily developed an overall bright red rash and the next day they went to the doctor. He prescribed antibiotics. Emily then developed severe asthma. She had had asthma previously 'but never anything as bad as this'. The medication seemed to make Emily's asthma worse and the next day she was medically evacuated to the nearest capital city with a collapsed lung.

The snack products contained three artificial colours (tartrazine, sunset yellow and chocolate brown), MSG and an antioxidant. All of these have been associated with both rash and asthma. Antibiotics and other medications in syrup form for children can contain artificial colour, artificial flavour and benzoate preservatives which can be associated with asthma. When a city doctor asked if Emily's asthma was related to anything she had eaten, Emily's mother said no.

Most asthmatics react to only one or two additives, some to more, but which ones? The failsafe diet will help you to find out what you need to avoid.

Patient Two

I came across Patient Two's (PT) case history in a medical journal. It is a perfect example of how a chronic asthmatic can be affected by a number of food chemicals without noticing, and how difficult it can be to sort out the effects of additives without a comprehensive elimination diet.

PT was a 23-year-old Australian nurse with a strong family history of asthma and had suffered from asthma since childhood. Wine was the only food product she had related to her asthma, although she had identified numerous airborne triggers. Until the age of 21, PT controlled her mild asthma well with preventers and relievers.

Over the next two years her asthma worsened into chronic, severe steroid-dependent asthma. PT needed many admissions to hospital. Four of these required ventilation. On the fifth, PT was admitted to hospital after two days of treating her increasing asthma at home with aggressive drug therapy. She was able to walk into the hospital emergency room where her condition was assessed as moderately severe. An hour after therapy began her condition deteriorated rapidly. PT was intubated and mechanically ventilated. Twelve hours later, while essentially wheeze-free, she was given an intravenous injection for nausea. Within minutes, she developed severe bronchospasm. Her previous hospital admissions revealed a similar pattern. She would arrive with moderately severe asthma and deteriorate rapidly when therapy began. Doctors suspected sensitivity to sulphite preservatives in drugs.

PT was put on an elimination diet and challenges were carried out in the intensive care ward. Peak flow rate—a test of lung function—was monitored for four to six hours after each challenge. She reacted to metabisulphite and benzoate preservatives, and to the colour tartrazine. When the tests were finished, PT went home and took an aspirin tablet for headache. Oops. The result was a severe asthma attack. Aspirin is a chemical called acetylsalicylic acid. Salicylates have been associated with asthma for a hundred years (see Chapter 7).

PT was put on an additive-free, low salicylate diet. Over the next six months her condition improved significantly. She was able to give up steroids and control her asthma with occasional medication. A few moderately severe attacks were easily controlled using a medication free of these preservatives. Then one fine morning PT was back in hospital—and the medical journals—fighting for her life. There was one more additive to be identified. You can read about PT's battle with MSG in the next chapter.

PT was lucky. She found doctors who knew about the effects of food additives and salicylates. Her life would have been very different otherwise. Medical journals contain accounts of asthmatics who are so ill they can't work, and even, sadly, coroners' reports of those who were unaware of this risk and didn't make it.

Remember, if your doctor doesn't know about the effects of food additives, you can find out for yourself.

6 Monosodium glutamate (MSG)

Summary
- MSG was introduced into food in America in 1948.
- The first adverse reaction to MSG was reported in 1968.
- The first asthmatic reaction to MSG was reported in 1981 by two Australian doctors.
- Since 1981, studies carried out by researchers supported by glutamate associations and studies carried out by independent researchers have reached opposite conclusions about the safety of MSG.
- Nearly 40 per cent of Melbourne asthmatic adults reported that food containing MSG affected their asthma.
- The only way to find out if you are affected by MSG is to test it for yourself.
- Asthmatics also need to regard with caution a new flavour enhancer (ribonucleotides, 635).

The first recorded reaction

The first recorded asthmatic reaction to MSG happened in 1981. It involved Patient Two (PT), the Australian nurse whose story was described in the last chapter. She had suffered many life-threatening asthma attacks, but when we last heard of her, she was doing well after six months on a diet free of sulphites, benzoates and artificial colours and low in salicylates.

Then one night PT went to a 15-course Chinese banquet. The next morning she developed severe asthma which would not respond to medication. She was admitted to hospital by 8 am and for the next three hours her asthma worsened despite treatment. By 11 am she was on mechanical ventilation with falling blood pressure and doctors fighting for her life. For five critical hours they used a partial cardiopulmonary bypass, until PT's blood pressure improved and she started recovering. Twenty-four hours later she could breathe by herself again. At that time it was unthinkable that an asthmatic could react to MSG so many hours after a meal. Six weeks later, PT ate a small Chinese meal and suffered an asthma attack the next morning.

To confirm that her reaction was due to MSG, PT bravely agreed to undergo a challenge with 2.5 grams of MSG. She was one of 32 asthmatic patients over three years whose reactions to MSG were challenged after two weeks on a comprehensive elimination diet. To try to recreate in the laboratory what had happened in the real world, PT was given her challenge at the same time that she had eaten her Chinese meals—at night. That night she remained asthma free. The next morning she developed severe acute asthma which required five hours of ventilator support, confirming the timing and severity of her previous reactions to MSG. For PT, this was the final piece of the asthma puzzle. Two years after identifying all her food triggers, her asthma was well controlled, she had stopped oral corticosteroids, rarely required admission to hospital and—a record for her—had not required ventilation in two years.

Altogether, 12 of the patients in the study reacted to MSG challenges with asthma. Some had noticed asthma after a Chinese meal. The others had not and were chosen for asthma which could not be stabilised with drug therapy. This study cannot be regarded as an indication of how many asthmatics react to MSG because it was not a random sample.

Researchers were particularly surprised by the long delayed reactions. Half of the reactions occurred six to 12 hours after the challenge. In general, people blame the food last eaten. A reaction which occurs more than half an hour later, and especially up to 12 hours later, would normally not be recognised as a food reaction. The exception to this rule occurs while people are undertaking an elimination diet, because then any reaction will be obvious. It was in this way that PT's reaction to MSG was first identified. The study was carried out by Drs David Allen, John Delohery and Gary Baker at the Royal North Shore Hospital in Sydney and published in a medical journal in 1987.

The MSG story

MSG occurs naturally in some foods like kombu seaweed, tomatoes and parmesan cheese. It was first isolated in 1908 by a professor at Tokyo University who became a partner in the Ajinomoto company, now a multi-billion dollar company providing more than half the world's MSG supply. As a concentrate MSG can easily be added to any foods in much greater quantities than in nature.

MSG did not become popular as an ingredient in American food until after World War II. Ironically, it had been noticed as an ingredient in Japanese army rations by US soldiers. Launched in the US in 1948 in a glittering symposium in Chicago, presided over by the Chief Quartermaster of the armed forces and attended by a who's who of the American food industry, MSG became a public relations triumph. The food industry embraced MSG and its use has increased forty-fold since then.

At first MSG was used mainly in Asian cooking in relatively large amounts, for example, 3 grams in a bowl of soup in a Chinese restaurant. It is now found in varying doses in virtually all soups, stocks, gravies, sauces, snack foods, takeaway and restaurant meals, including fried chicken and pizza. Flavour sachets in products such as instant noodles and crisps are particularly high in MSG. Although Westerners assume that MSG consumption is high in Asian countries, estimates of average MSG intake found extreme users in the UK consumed more than those in Japan or Korea. By definition, extreme users consume three times the average. They had an average intake of 16 grams of MSG per week—not counting snacks and foods consumed outside the home which would clearly be a major source of MSG. The consumption of MSG by 15–25 year olds was considerably higher than the rest of the population.

No free lunch

The first reactions to MSG were identified in 1968 by a Dr Robert Kwok who had emigrated from China to the US. Dr Kwok reported that although he never had the problem in China, about 20 minutes into a meal at certain Chinese restaurants he suffered numbness, tingling and tightness of the chest that lasted approximately two hours. This collection of symptoms became known as Chinese Restaurant Syndrome.

A year after Dr Kwok reported his symptoms, researchers in the US found that everyone will react to MSG if the dose is high enough. Every day, 36 subjects ate chicken soup with added MSG. The doses increased slowly. Half of the subjects reacted to doses between 1.5 and 4 grams. Most of the rest reacted to doses between 5 and 12 grams. Researchers commented that it would be possible to prepare a meal containing 10–12 grams of MSG per person by following the manufacturer's recommendations. Other researchers have remarked that it is possible to consume that amount in a Chinese banquet. In that study researchers were only looking for the traditional Chinese restaurant reactions of burning, facial pressure and chest pain, although in other studies they noted migraine, gastric distress and a doctor who admitted himself to hospital, convinced he was experiencing the symptoms of a heart attack—typically pain in the chest, tingling and numbness from the chest down the left arm and a feeling of impending doom.

Defenders of the faith

In response to the possibility of MSG having toxic potential, a number of associations were organised. The International Glutamate Technical Committee (IGTC)—formed in 1969—consists of doctors and scientists who meet once a year, with secretariat provided by Ajinomoto, to sponsor MSG research.

The *Glutamate Association* was established in 1977 to provide communication and awareness on the 'use and safety of glutamates' (www.msgfacts.com).

The *International Glutamate Information Service* (IGIS) provides information about glutamates based on 'scientific evidence which confirms the safety and the benefits of this widely used food ingredient' (www.glutamate.org). It is supported by the *Australian Glutamate Information Service*.

Other non-profit organisations which offer science-based information are encouraged to pass on information from the Glutamate Association. An award-winning science website at the University of Texas recommends the *International Food Information Council* (IFIC) website guides. 'A source of good information,' it says, while warning that 'they take a definitely pro-industry stance and tend to gloss over areas of nutritional or food safety debate: for instance, they argue that monosodium glutamate is a perfectly safe food additive.'

Allergists, dietitians and nutritionists appear to have been particularly targeted. Glutamate industry involvement is rarely obvious. That's what makes it so effective.

Numbers wars

In 1976 a survey found that 25 per cent of the population experience adverse reactions after a meal in a Chinese restaurant. This study was funded in part by a grant from the National Eye Institute, interested because MSG had been found to cause retinal damage in newborn animals.

In 1979 a market research questionnaire (commissioned by Ajinomoto) found that less than 2 per cent of the population suffer from Chinese Restaurant Syndrome after a meal. I suspect this lower figure was achieved because the study did not include reactions which occurred outside a given time limit and narrow symptom range. Soon after this study, the US Food and Drug Administration (FDA) started quoting the figure that only 2 per cent of the population react to MSG.

The battle for statistical high ground had begun. It is in any food industry's best interests if only a small number of people are seen to react to their product. So when PT and the others in that study came along with their asthmatic reaction to MSG, glutamate supporters must have felt threatened. Then something happened which made it important for them to prove that MSG does not provoke asthma.

MSG goes to court

As an asthmatic, Californian businessman David Livingston knows he reacts to MSG so he avoids it. In July 1993, Livingston went to a Marie Callender's restaurant for a business lunch. He told the waitress he had asthma and wanted to know if the vegetable soup contained MSG. The waitress assured him the soup was 'made from the freshest ingredients, from scratch . . . every day'. It was later found to contain a 'beef base' which had MSG clearly listed on the label.

On the way back to the office, Livingston felt an asthma attack coming on. When his inhaler failed to provide relief, he drove immediately to his primary care physician, five minutes away. There he suffered an anaphylactic reaction including respiratory arrest. CPR was initiated and continued in an ambulance but after reaching hospital Livingstone went into full cardiac arrest and was without pulse for seven minutes. He was finally resuscitated and remained unconscious on a respirator in the Intensive Care Unit for three days. He remained a further three days in the hospital for observation and treatment. As a result of lack of oxygen, Livingston suffered brain damage and remains with a slight neurological deficit. One year later, David Livingston initiated a lawsuit against Marie Callender's Inc.

At about that time, researchers Drs Ronald Simon, Donald Stevenson and Katharine Woessner at the Scripps Research Institute and Scripps Clinic began a study supported by the IGTC. As a result, two papers were published, which seemed to demolish the idea that MSG could be connected with asthma. Or did they?

Selection of subjects

Consumer groups first heard of the study when an advertisement appeared in the *Los Angeles Times* seeking test subjects for a new asthma study at the Scripps. One MSG-sensitive woman who replied was told that '(1) if she feared her asthma reactions to be serious that she should not apply for the study, (2) that the person who was screening the applicants didn't believe that MSG could cause asthma reactions, and (3) that she was most likely responding to sulphites, and not to MSG'. This was reported in the newsletter of the No MSG group.

I think this is a good illustration of how double blinded placebo-control (DBPC) studies could be biased, despite DBPC protocols. By rejecting asthmatics who think they react to MSG, can't you be pretty sure to run a study with no reactors?

The study tested 100 asthmatic subjects (30 subjects with 'a history of Oriental restaurant asthma attacks' and 70 with a negative history). There were no signs or symptoms of asthma related to MSG. However:

- there is a question mark over the selection of subjects;
- absence of evidence is not evidence of absence; and
- the study did not use a comprehensive elimination diet.

The study ended with the conclusion that 'it is important to maintain a healthy scepticism about the existence of MSG sensitivity in individuals with asthma'. A year later, DD Stevenson published a review about MSG and asthma, seriously criticising the Australian doctors' study of MSG-induced asthma.

The full story of the relationship between Drs Simon and Stevenson and the glutamate industry is discussed in an article, 'A study in suppression of information', by Dr Adrienne Samuels published in the journal *Accountability in Research* (available on the internet at www.truthinlabeling.org/1-manuscript.htm).

The verdict

In July 1997, David Livingston went to court against Marie Callender's Inc. Dr Simon from the Scripps was called as an expert witness in the court case. You can read about his testimony at www.truthinlabeling.org/scripps1.

Mr Livingston's strict liability claim was dismissed on the ground that there was nothing wrong with the soup, or the MSG in the soup. At an application for appeal in March 1999, the matter was remanded for a retrial, on the issue of whether any defendant is liable for 'failure to warn of an ingredient to which a substantial number of the population are allergic' and 'the ingredient . . . is one which the consumer would reasonably not expect to find in the product . . .' You can read this court report at http://caselaw.findlaw.com.data2/californiastatecases/b115078.pdf.

How to recognise an industry supported researcher

You can find studies about monosodium glutamate in the Medline medical database at www.pubmed.com. Keep in mind that 13 of the world's top medical journals imposed rules regarding disclosure of company ties in 2001. Here are some hints from Dr Samuels about how to recognise the influence of industry in research or public talks:

- Researchers will claim MSG is safe.
- They will refer to studies as 'randomised double blind cross-over design' which gives the casual reader the impression

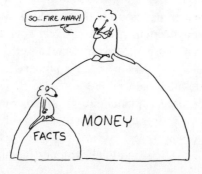

that subjects were drawn randomly from the general population—in fact, subjects are often carefully selected.
- Conclusions will not follow from the results in the study.
- Critics of MSG will be disparaged or made the subject of jokes—critics don't report adverse reactions, they 'complain'.
- Jokey generalisations are presented in serious papers—'if you eat too much of anything you'll get sick'.
- Existing data may be distorted or trivialised.
- Reports of human suffering are dismissed as anecdotes.
- Inaccurate generalisations will be presented by alleged authorities—'monosodium glutamate has been used in the orient for more than 2000 years' (it was only synthesised in 1902).

By now, you might be wondering, as I was, why don't the people in charge do something about this? Dr Samuels' answer is that the influence of the glutamate industry 'can be felt at every level'.

Pressure on the media

Negative mention of MSG by the major media sources has been virtually non-existent since *60 Minutes* in the US aired a story about the toxic effects of MSG in 1991. Don Hewett of *60 Minutes* said on television that he had never had so much pressure applied to him by industry as he had prior to the MSG segment going to air. Dr Samuels comments that although rated by TV guides as one of the two most watched segments of the year, *60 Minutes* now won't touch a story about MSG.

How many?

So how many asthmatics do react to MSG? We don't know. What we do know is that:
- some asthmatics are affected by MSG
- some people are more sensitive than others
- effects are related to dose
- children are more vulnerable to the effects of additives than adults.

WHAT THE RESEARCHERS SAY
Independent
- 'This study suggests that MSG is not safe for some individuals with asthma,' Allen and others, 1987
- 'Two patients presented with mild bronchospasm, occurring 6 to 10 hours after the ingestion [of 2.5 gm of MSG].' Moneret–Vautrin, 1987
- 'After one month on the elimination diet, food chemical challenge caused [11 asthmatic reactions, including] one to MSG.' Hodge and others, 1996

Glutamate association (IGTC) supported
- 'It is important to maintain a healthy scepticism about the existence of MSG sensitivity in individuals with asthma,' Woessner and others, 1999
- 'The existence of MSG–induced asthma . . . has not been established conclusively.' Stevenson, 2000

Publication sponsored by the International Glutamate Information Service
- 'Adults with asthma do not need to restrict MSG intake.' Woods, 2001

What the Melbourne adults say

Remember the adult asthmatics in Melbourne who were asked which foods affected them? Nearly 40 per cent reported asthma after consuming MSG. A study was organised to test this perception.

Twelve of the asthmatics who thought they were MSG-sensitive followed an elimination diet—not the one I recommend—for two weeks, before taking capsule challenges of MSG (1 and 5 grams) and placebo. The results looked like what you get when you don't use an adequate elimination diet. There were 15 reactions in 8 subjects including false negatives (reacting to small doses of MSG but not to large doses), false positives and lots of placebo reactions. The one subject who did react to both MSG doses did not react significantly.

When results are mixed like this, it means that a stable

baseline—against which reactions may be seen—has not been established. Perhaps the diet didn't exclude enough food chemicals, or wasn't followed strictly enough, or for long enough.

The researchers, led by Dr Rosalie Woods, concluded that MSG-induced asthma was not demonstrated in this study. I agree. However, the study did not prove the non-existence of MSG-induced asthma. I disagree with Dr Woods' conclusion in a later review, see box on previous page.

How necessary is it?

MSG is an unnecessary additive. Our grandparents lived their whole lives without adding it to their foods. Children in Saudi Arabian villages don't eat it. Its benefits are to make cheap or inferior ingredients taste irresistible. The glutamate industry promotes it as an appetite enhancer for the elderly. The elderly are vulnerable to the effects of food additives because their livers and kidneys become less efficient at detoxifying chemicals. Distressed seniors attend my talks or write to me in laborious longhand asking about reactions like a swollen tongue, asthma and anginal pain which isn't angina, after certain meals (Me: Which meals? DS: Well, when I make stir-fry . . . Me: Do you add any seasoning? DS: Well, yes, I do . . .). They are more than happy to avoid MSG. In western countries facing an epidemic of obesity, who needs an appetite enhancer which makes you eat more?

Oh no, not *another* flavour enhancer . . .

A new flavour enhancer called ribonucleotides (additive 635) has been slowly introduced into our food supply over about the last five years. It is a combination of sodium guanylate (627) and sodium inosinate (631).

I first heard about this additive shortly after it was introduced. A paediatrician sent me a list of ingredients in instant noodles and asked which one could cause a dramatic skin rash. A few weeks later, a two-year-old girl who had instant noodles every night for dinner ate a different brand and developed a rash so severe she was taken to the emergency room in the middle of the night and spent two weeks on antihistamines. The only difference between brands was the inclusion of ribonucleotides.

I have received many similar reports of severe itchy rash from 6 to 30 hours later. Because the reaction is delayed, many people do not realise the cause of the rash. It can be accompanied by life-threatening swelling of the lips, throat and tongue, and asthmatics can suffer breathing difficulties. One schoolboy was 'minutes from death' by the time he got to a doctor's surgery after eating a pie, yet a few chips resulted in only the rash.

There are three unusual characteristics of reactions to this additive:

- people always say they have never had a reaction like it before;
- there seems to be a very fine line between no reaction at all and a severe reaction, for example, people who can manage one packet of flavoured chips may react badly to slightly more than one packet of the same chips;
- the rash can take a long time—two weeks or more—to clear up.

See for yourself

Consumers say they are affected by MSG. Glutamate associations say they are not. We have seen that the effects of food additives are consistently underestimated. We know that some asthmatics are affected by MSG. If MSG contributes to your asthma, it is important for you to know. You can find out for yourself whether MSG affects you, see p. 170. If it does, you can follow the directions on p. 193, How to avoid MSG.

7 Salicylates and amines

Summary
- Salicylates are found in aspirin, other non-steroidal anti-inflammatory drugs (NSAIDs) and plant foods including most fruit and some vegetables.
- Asthmatics are often unaware of their sensitivity to salicylates.
- Salicylates are also found in toothpaste, lotions, pollen and fragrances.
- Aspirin-induced asthma (Samter's syndrome) consists of asthma, sensitivity to aspirin, rhinitis or nasal polyps and sometimes urticaria.
- Salicylates may affect 20 per cent or more of all asthmatics.
- The salicylate content of foods in the West is probably increasing through plant breeding and some genetic engineering.
- Salicylates are not the only naturally occurring food chemicals which can affect asthmatics. Amines and natural glutamates can cause problems too.
- Other healthy foods which can cause problems include wheat, gluten and dairy foods.
- There is no risk—and a big potential benefit—associated with going additive free. If you want to exclude healthy foods in the long term, the link with your asthma should be confirmed, and your nutrition should be checked.

Aspirin and salicylates

After sulphites, salicylates in drugs and foods are probably the most important group of chemicals affecting asthmatics. As with additives, the effects of these chemicals are not a true allergy. Although many asthmatics have never heard of them, nearly 20 per cent of the Melbourne survey group reported that they were avoiding salicylates.

The best known of the salicylate family is aspirin. The name salicylate comes from salix, meaning willow, because aspirin was first extracted from the bark of the willow tree. When it was introduced in 1898, aspirin was hailed as a wonder drug free of side effects but reports of aspirin-induced asthma, anaphylaxis and hives began almost immediately. Salicylates are also present in other non-steroidal anti-inflammatory drugs (NSAIDs) and are natural components of plant foods including most fruit and some vegetables.

How do you know if you react?

People assume that they will know if they are sensitive to aspirin because they will have seen a reaction, but as with additives, this is true only for the minority.

To test whether asthmatics were aware of aspirin sensitivity, researchers at the Scripps Clinic in California asked asthmatic patients if their asthma was triggered by aspirin. Patients who thought they didn't react to aspirin or weren't sure were asked to take part in a study. They were given a disguised aspirin tablet and observed. Nearly 20 per cent of the group reacted. Researchers noticed a very important difference between those who had recognised their sensitivity and those who hadn't:

- all of the asthmatics who knew they reacted to aspirin *reacted within 10–20 minutes.*
- all of the asthmatics who had said they didn't react to aspirin, or 'not sure', *reacted at least 45 minutes later and in some cases, many hours later.*

It is the same old story. People who have quick, strong reactions will notice their sensitivity, but most won't. That doesn't mean they're not affected. Continual exposure can result in chronic lung inflammation and asthma which comes and goes without an obvious cause.

NSAIDs can be dangerous

Reactions to aspirin can be life threatening. Even more worrying is the increasing variety of salicylate-containing NSAIDs such as ibuprofen. Consumers, and even experts, don't always know which drugs contain salicylates.

Aspirin sensitivity is a sign that patients shouldn't take NSAIDs. I have heard pharmacists ask customers, 'Are you an asthmatic? If you are sensitive to aspirin, it's not a good idea to take this medication . . .'. 'I don't know,' the customer often says, 'I don't think so.' But they might be like the late reactors in the study on the previous page.

Death from a NSAID

Appearing in the medical journals is a procession of people of all ages whose stories are told as case histories. Many of them are dramatic or triumphant or tragic. One of the saddest I've come across was a man from New York with a twisted ankle (TA).

TA had developed asthma at the age of 49. He was 55 when he twisted his ankle. At the hospital, he was given a prescription for naproxen for pain relief and sent home. About an hour after he took a naproxen tablet he developed difficulty breathing. His wife gave him some asthma medication (a theophylline tablet) and went to make a coffee which had helped in the past. When she returned TA was unconscious. He died in the ambulance on the way to hospital.

Even in the official jargon from the county coroner, you could tell that everyone was stunned by TA's sudden death. TA had two risk factors for aspirin-induced asthma—asthma which begins in the 30s or 40s and a history of nasal polyps, although salicylate intolerance can equally occur without these.

'We should educate patients to eliminate the risk posed by NSAIDs and other agents that may induce asthma attacks,' say medical researchers at the University of Fujita in Japan. As an asthmatic, unless you have done an elimination diet and passed your salicylate challenge, you do not know whether you are salicylate sensitive. Approach aspirin and NSAIDs with caution. Either use alternative medication, or have someone with you when you take it. You are not necessarily going to react the first time, see p. 140.

Salicylates in foods

Most plants manufacture salicylic acid, in varying amounts, as a natural pesticide to protect themselves against insects and diseases. Everyone knows that man-made pesticides can cause health problems in humans but there is little awareness of the effects of salicylates.

An analysis of the salicylate contents of fruit, vegetables, herbs and spices found prunes and gherkins were the highest in salicylates. Common very high-salicylate foods included tomatoes, especially concentrated in puree, sauce or juice, oranges especially juice, and grapes, especially wine, sultanas and raisins. Low-salicylate foods included wheat, rice, pears, potatoes and beans. A previous food list, used in the well-known Feingold diet for hyperactive children, had been calculated in 1901. It was less comprehensive and omitted such high-salicylate foods as pineapple.

Salicylates in toothpaste

Peppermint is very high in salicylates. A British study of the effects of food on asthmatic children found reactions to peppermint and honey but dismissed these as 'unimportant foods'. Both are high in salicylates. Peppermint is actually very important indeed.

Thirteen per cent of asthmatics in the Melbourne survey reported toothpaste as triggering their asthma. There are three papers reporting toothpaste-flavour-induced asthma, including the case of a Japanese teenager whose asthma developed at the age of 15. She noticed a sensitivity to toothpaste. Her sensitivity to salicylates was confirmed two years later when she suffered loss of consciousness after taking a salicylate-containing analgesic for a common cold.

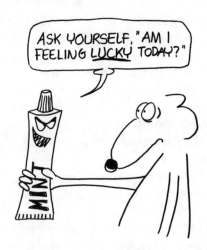

Those of us who work with children's behavioural problems know that the wrong toothpaste alone can overcome the benefits of the failsafe diet. Coloured toothpaste can cause problems but if the toothpaste is white then flavour is the likely cause of the reaction. Herbal toothpastes also contain salicylates. It is possible to buy white unflavoured toothpaste and there are alternatives (p. 239).

Salicylates in liniments and fragrance

Salicylates can be absorbed through the skin from oil of winter-green in liniments and oils for muscle aches and pains and can cause severe reactions in asthmatics. Salicylates in teething gel can affect babies. Inhaled salicylates in menthol, various pollens like birch pollen, and fragrances such as wintergreen in soap and cosmetics are a similar hazard for the very sensitive (pp. 86–8).

Samter's syndrome

One of the medical researchers who was instrumental in dis-covering the effects of salicylates on asthma was the great Dr Max Samter. Smuggled out of Germany as a child during World War I and deafened by a shell explosion in Okinawa in World War II, Dr Samter turned to research. A major discovery of his was a special kind of asthma in which asthma, aspirin-sensitivity and nasal polyps were always present—now known as Samter's Syndrome.

This syndrome is thought to affect about 3 per cent of asthmatic patients in general, and 20 per cent of patients with severe asthma. The early stages are bronchial asthma and rhinitis. Onset is usually in the 30s and 40s age group and more women are affected than men. Intolerance to aspirin can develop suddenly at any age.

Ironically, Dr Samter ultimately decided that low salicylate diets were a waste of time because he saw so many patients fall ill while following strictly what was thought to be a low salicylate diet. He died before he could realise it was the incomplete salicylate list itself, not the concept of the low-salicylate diet, that was at fault.

> I have Samter's syndrome and for the last 29 years, I have been taking medications and trying to stay alive. When I found the Australian salicylate lists I was so excited. I could finally understand what was happening. I was inadvertently eating salicylates every day.
> —*Reader from the US*

How many react?

The new salicylate food lists from research conducted in 1985 are used in the failsafe diet recommended in this book (p. 219). They were also used in the Children's Hospital study (see p. 23). More than 20 per cent of the children reacted to salicylates. The asthmatic adults in the Melbourne survey also reported 20 per cent—one in five.

These figures suggest that the role of salicylates in asthma should be taken seriously. Conditions other than asthma have also been linked to salicylates in Royal Prince Alfred Hospital (RPAH) studies—approximately 50 per cent of people with food-related eczema, and 70 per cent of people with food-related irritable bowel, headache or ADHD symptoms react to salicylates.

Effects of the failsafe diet

In the Children's Hospital study, the six children who reacted to salicylates went on the failsafe diet for three months. Only one child—a chronic asthmatic—fully complied with the diet. His improvement was dramatic. In three months his asthma improved, he showed improved lung function and was able to be weaned off oral steroids. Doctors concluded that treating by diet is too hard. I don't agree. Every day I see families doing this diet with difficult children.

A low salicylate diet for adults

For motivated adults, the failsafe diet is usually considered to be easy. A young woman I'll call Rosemary developed severe asthma which was not controlled by drugs. Rosemary was admitted to hospital about once a month with life-threatening asthma attacks. As a last resort she tried the elimination diet but soon ended up in hospital again.

A hospital dietitian realised that Rosemary had somehow mixed up the instructions regarding the elimination diet. Instead of eating from the 'foods to eat' list, she had been eating the 'foods to avoid'. When that was sorted out, Rosemary's asthma improved. She was sensitive to salicylates.

Lisa's baby

Salicylates are unfair. People who eat junk food know they are making bad choices. But salicylates are in healthy food. Lisa was a sole parent, breastfeeding her baby and eating home-grown organic whole food, honey instead of sugar, brown bread, vegetarian, healthiest-diet-possible foods. By the time he was 13 months old her son had been hospitalised for a week with severe asthma and was on daily medication.

Looking for an alternative, Lisa discovered the failsafe diet. As soon as she saw the list of salicylate-containing foods she realised what the problem was. Lisa and her baby had been eating a diet exceptionally high in salicylates.

Salicylates around the world

My family has been on a low salicylate diet for eight years. When we left Australia recently for a six-month trip around the world, I really didn't know how we were going to cope with the food.

Within days of arriving in our first destination, the island of Bali in Indonesia, we realised that the local diet was virtually failsafe. Of course we avoided Western-style processed foods like additive-laden jam, fruit juice and Western-style fast food. Eating such simple Balinese foods as rice, fresh fish, chicken, eggs, stir-fried low to moderate salicylate vegetables and local fruit, we soon noticed we could eat many more fruits and vegetables than were possible at home.

As our trip progressed through developing countries like Nepal, India and Egypt we even enjoyed normally disastrous high salicylate foods like apricots, tomatoes, dates, strawberries and curries.

The varieties we were eating were local, small, usually home-grown traditional fruits and vegetables. They were picked ripe and were best eaten that day or the next. They had poor keeping qualities and squashed easily but tasted sweet and delicious and didn't affect us. We wondered why. It is possible there are a number of factors involved. Could it be that we were more relaxed and on holidays, I wondered at first, but as soon as we arrived back in a country with a Western lifestyle it became clear that wasn't the case.

Some other possibilities were a much lower total load of chemicals like pesticides, household cleaners, and fragrances, or plants grown in a climate which was more naturally suited to them than the harsh Australian environment. Also, in traditional villages, companion planting occurs naturally. Each little garden has a mixture of fruits, vegetables, herbs, flowers and other foods. Plants grown in a companion planting environment are probably a lot less stressed and therefore may develop fewer salicylates. I don't know which of these answers is correct— maybe all of them. What I do know is that for three months it was very pleasant to be in cultures where we could walk into any restaurant and eat anything, knowing that the traditional foods would not contribute to any of the Western diseases of affluence.

The Western diet and salicylates

After several months in developing countries, we arrived in Europe. Within a week, we had noticed the difference. Not only are fruits and vegetables grown for Western markets higher in salicylates but the Western diet is also much higher in salicylate-containing foods. In traditional cultures fruits and vegetables are eaten mainly fresh and unprocessed. In Egypt when we had orange juice, it was not from a strong concentrate but at fresh fruit stalls where four small sweet oranges would be pressed into a glass as we watched. Tomatoes would be served fresh, soft, red and ripe as part of the salad.

In the West, and particularly in English-speaking countries, fruits are presented as highly concentrated juices or fruit flavours in a multitude of processed foods from breakfast cereals to yoghurts to cookies and fruit bars and other snacks. High-salicylate vegetable concentrate such as tomato paste is added to nearly everything to increase flavour. In traditional cultures, we ate lower-salicylate fruits and tomatoes in small quantities. As the ISAAC studies found, in traditional diets, the majority of calories come from low-salicylate sources like rice, bread or chapattis.

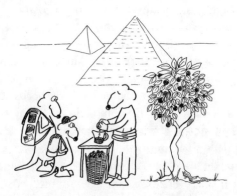

Plant breeding

During the last hundred years, fruits, vegetables and cereal crops in the West have undergone major changes, and it hasn't been an accident. People are concerned about genetic engineering, but modification of our food has been happening for decades in a process called plant breeding.

Plant breeders select whichever varieties are the most successful for a natural resistance to pests or suitability for packing, storage and transport. These traits are then encouraged through selective breeding. Any other side effects that happen are ignored.

Since salicylates are natural pesticides which result in better resistance to pests and diseases, plants in the west have almost certainly been bred for increasingly higher salicylate content. Plants that are firm and unripe are higher in salicylates, but easier to transport. You can see why varieties like that would be chosen for supermarkets.

Genetic engineering can accelerate this process. Right now, in Holland, a team of agricultural scientists at Leiden University are developing high-salicylate wheats and rice through genetic engineering. If they succeed in releasing these cereals worldwide, salicylate levels in our food supply will rise yet again. There will be fewer safe foods. More people will reach a level at which they are noticeably affected. Asthmatics who react to salicylates will need yet more medication.

The National Asthma Council acknowledges the effects of dietary salicylates on asthma. They suggest that the addition of a leukotriene receptor antagonist such as montelukast to your existing medication regime may improve asthma control. Side-effects are a possibility with any drug, see p. 109. You may prefer to eliminate the cause of the problem rather than to treat the symptoms.

Salicylates aren't the only ones

There are two other categories of naturally occurring food chemicals which may cause problems for asthmatics. Natural glutamates in tasty cheeses, tomatoes, wine and other foods have already been mentioned in the last chapter. The doses of these chemicals in natural foods are much smaller than can be added in a concentrated form, but for some sensitive people that can be enough to cause problems.

Amines are naturally occurring chemicals which are strongly associated with migraines but can also affect asthmatics. Traditional high amine foods linked to migraines are chocolate and cheese. Amines are the breakdown products of protein and so are also found in foods like aged meat and frozen or processed seafoods. There is a list of foods containing salicylates, amines and natural glutamates on pp. 219–31.

With food intolerance, anything can happen. I know asthmatics whose elimination diet showed up sensitivity to wheat or gluten (see p. 209). And then, of course, there are dairy foods which are covered in the next chapter. There is no risk, and a potentially big benefit, from going additive-free, but healthy foods are another story. Asthmatics should not exclude healthy foods from their diet without confirming the culprits, and checking their diet with a nutritionist.

8 Dairy foods

Summary
- The association between asthma and dairy products is a hot topic. Asthmatics say dairy products affect them; the National Asthma Council says dairy foods are unlikely to affect asthmatics.
- More asthmatics say that dairy foods affect them than any other food but studies suggest that dairy foods are less likely to trigger asthma than food additives—especially sulphites—and salicylates.
- Dairy foods can affect asthma through either *food allergy* or *food intolerance*. Only about 2 per cent of asthmatics are affected by a true milk allergy.
- Intolerance reactions to dairy foods are more difficult to identify because they are usually delayed by 20 hours or more. People who respond like this are likely to have chronic ill health and multiple food intolerances.
- It is possible to misinterpret food reactions unless you use a skinprick test for allergy and an elimination diet for intolerances.
- Dairy foods may be associated with other health problems which bother asthmatics such as frequent ear infections, hayfever and loose cough.
- Dairy foods are an important source of nutrients and should not be avoided unnecessarily. If you think you react to milk, you should confirm the reaction. This is particularly important for asthmatics since commonly used asthma medications may be associated with bone loss.

The association between asthma and dairy products is controversial. Some asthmatics say dairy products affect them more than any other food. Dairy products were the most commonly avoided foods in the Melbourne survey of asthmatic adults. Of those who reported reactions to food, nearly 40 per cent reported a reaction to dairy. Similarly, a survey in New Zealand found nearly 80 per cent of asthmatic children had been or were avoiding dairy products. Again, dairy products were clearly the biggest category of avoided foods.

The Australian National Asthma Council (NAC) does not consider cow's milk allergy to be a common cause of asthma. This is true, although we also need to consider the effects of food intolerance. Studies have shown that only about 2 per cent of asthmatics have cow's milk allergy—a lot less than asthmatic responders to sulphites and other food chemicals. True allergy to cow's milk is more likely to cause rashes or diarrhoea than asthma, but for asthmatics who are affected, milk allergy is important. Babies with a family history of food allergies, eczema, asthma and hayfever are the most likely to develop food allergies themselves. With a true milk allergy, there will be an obvious reaction to a dairy food within 30 minutes of consumption, although if dairy foods are eaten frequently, the relationship may be hidden.

True milk allergy: Richard's story

When Richard was born 20 years ago, he had many relatives with allergies and asthma so his mother followed the recommendations for allergic babies. She breastfed for twelve months, and delayed introduction of known allergens like cow's milk and eggs. Richard suffered from frequent ear infections and had a sensitive stomach.

His first asthma attack, at the age of two-and-a-half, hospitalised him for a week. He rapidly became a chronic severe asthmatic needing daily medication. Skinprick tests showed he was allergic to 'nearly everything'. Cutting out cow's milk didn't seem to help.

It wasn't until a naturopath suggested avoidance of *all* dairy foods including butter, icecream, cream, skim milk and whey powder in processed foods like bread and biscuits that Richard's mother was able to see a connection—Richard would have an asthma attack half an hour after ingesting any form of dairy food. At the same time that he developed asthma, Richard became 'overactive'. His behaviour was worsened by asthma medication.

By the time he was four, Richard was on a strict additive-free, dairy-free diet. His only asthma attacks were on the rare occasions that he ate dairy foods. Between the ages of 12 and 18, Richard stuck to his family's diet and thought he had grown out of his asthma. When he went to university Richard started eating anything he wanted. His asthma returned and he now takes daily preventer and reliever medication.

An allergy–intolerance mix

It is possible to have a mixture of food allergies and food intolerances, and although most children with allergies are only allergic to one or two foods, for them allergy to both cow's milk and soy is relatively common. An elimination diet will help to sort out the culprits when many foods are involved, as this nurse from Victoria reports:

> My youngest son was diagnosed with asthma at nine months. He is now three. He has had a wheeze from three weeks old and been on puffers and preventers all his short life, until starting on the elimination diet. Of what I've challenged so far, any time he has dairy, soy products and sulphites, his wheeze starts again. We now use a calcium fortified rice milk.

Asthma as an intolerance reaction to cow's milk

Compared to true allergic or IgE reactions, intolerance reactions to dairy foods are much more difficult to identify because they are usually very delayed. In a series of long-term studies at Melbourne's Children's Hospital, Dr David Hill realised that some people are late responders, usually reacting more than 20 hours and up to several days after ingestion of normal volumes of cow's milk. They are likely to develop bronchial symptoms, diarrhoea or eczema in any combination. Late reactors generally have a history of chronic ill health such as irritable bowel symptoms and multiple food intolerance.

Sarah's story: a late reactor

Sarah is a nurse who developed adult onset asthma after the birth of her first child. At first she noticed that viruses resulted in chest congestion which would last for weeks. This gradually worsened. Although she never experienced life-threatening asthma, she had daily chest discomfort and was diagnosed with asthma. She used a puffer daily and eventually also daily steroid puffers. Ten years later the whole family embarked on the elimination diet for their eldest child's behaviour. Sarah immediately noticed an improvement in her chronic stomach discomfort. After six months on the elimination diet, the family also started avoiding dairy foods.

Soon Sarah realised that she no longer had asthmatic symptoms so she stopped taking prophylactic medication. In the years that have followed Sarah has mostly avoided the foods which affect her. Through occasional inadvertent challenges she has noticed that her asthma is triggered by sulphites 12 hours after eating sausages or a large quantity of dried fruit, benzoates in diet cola, and dairy foods. Although she eats dairy products only as a treat, if she has a large amount of icecream—or any dairy product—she will get asthma the next day.

Since changing what she eats, Sarah has noticed the biggest change is her ability to recover quickly from viruses. She says, 'Before I stopped dairy foods, if I developed a respiratory problem of some sort, despite prophylaxis it would drag on for weeks.' Now when she gets a viral infection, she only sometimes needs a puffer. Very occasionally, if that is not enough, she will use a short-term burst of prophylactics which quickly solves the problem.

The NAC and dairy

The NAC recommendation on allergy, below, with fail to catch late responders like Sarah. After a survey showed that nearly 10 per cent of GPs will recommend patients with asthma decrease their intake of dairy food, the NAC, together with the Australian Dairy Corporation, began a program of doctor education. Under both logos, they sent a letter to GPs stating that

> The National Asthma Campaign recommends dairy foods as part of a balanced diet for asthma patients. Dairy foods provide essential nutrients and should not be avoided by asthma patients unless an allergy has been firmly established; asthma reactions to dairy products are unlikely to occur.

Alfred Hospital, Melbourne, study

The link between asthma and non-allergic reactions to dairy products was tested in a small study at Melbourne's Alfred Hospital.

The study involved 10 asthmatics who thought milk triggered their asthma and 10 who didn't. Researchers chose subjects who were not allergic to milk as shown by a skin prick test. This was a study of intolerance, not allergy. The subjects agreed before the study that they would react to a glass of milk within hours although this is not an appropriate challenge—intolerance reactions to milk are usually delayed, up to 20 hours or more, and build up slowly. It is possible that these subjects had never done an elimination diet before and didn't realise how they would react under those conditions. In fact, 20 per cent of the subjects did react, but with symptoms like blocked nose which may have been the beginning of a reaction but were dismissed by researchers as not 'convincing'. The study concluded that 'it is unlikely dairy products have a specific bronchoconstrictor effect in most patients with asthma, regardless of their perceptions'. This is a very big conclusion for a little study. A more appropriate conclusion from this particular study is that some patients' perceptions of cow's milk as an asthma trigger may be

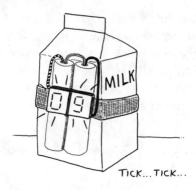

TICK... TICK...

mistaken although a better challenge would have been 1–3 glasses of cow's milk every day for a week.

Failsafe asthmatics who are sensitive to milk are angry about this study. 'But I wouldn't have reacted that quickly,' said one. 'Don't they know about delayed reactions?' It is the same old confusion about the effects of food allergy and food intolerance as described on p. 8.

Food reactions can be misinterpreted

It is possible to misinterpret the effects of foods especially when the reaction is delayed. Remember Robert on p. 23? His asthma cleared up when he did the elimination diet for irritable bowel symptoms. One night he broke his diet by eating preserved sausages. The next day his mother reported, 'He had asthma this morning after breakfast. He hasn't had that for a while. It can't have been anything he ate, he had the same breakfast as usual.' Then she decided, 'It must have been the milk.' But Robert ate his breakfast with milk every morning throughout the diet with no asthma. He had broken the diet the night before for the first time by eating sausages which are a common source of sulphites. Asthmatic reactions to sulphites can be delayed by 12 hours or more. Robert's asthma was almost certainly triggered by the sulphites in the sausages rather than the milk on his breakfast, but people forget and tend to blame the food last eaten.

It is also possible to be misled by improvements. When avoiding a certain food, you may have removed other provoking chemicals as well, for example, salicylates as well as dairy foods in strawberry yoghurt. The moral of this story is: if you think your asthma is affected by dairy foods, depending on whether you have a family history of allergy or intolerance, have a skin prick test or do an elimination diet with a dairy challenge (p. 171) to make certain. It is not enough to cut out a food and feel better.

Does milk make mucus?

There are other conditions which may increase the discomfort of asthma. One woman whose asthma was triggered by preservatives and MSG wrote 'while dairy doesn't provoke an asthma attack in me, it definitely increases mucus and causes post nasal drip, among other things, which are not helpful with asthma'.

The Flinders University mucus study

The NAC says that 'there is no medical foundation for the widely held view that dairy products increase mucus secretions'. In the entire Medline medical database, only one group of researchers has investigated the 'milk makes mucus' idea. At Flinders University, 60 volunteers were exposed to a cold virus. To measure nasal secretions, researchers asked volunteers to put their tissues in a sealed plastic bag immediately after blowing their noses. After weighing the tissues for 10 days, researchers found no difference between those consuming dairy foods and those not, although the volunteers who believed that dairy foods affected them reported more cough and congestion.

Hayfever

Allergic rhinitis, also known as hayfever, is characterised by sneezing, running or blocked nose and watering eyes. Up to 80 per cent of asthmatics suffer hayfever and 30–40 per cent of people with hayfever have asthma. I was one of them until I changed my diet. Challenges revealed that, for me, my hayfever is associated with a combination of dairy products and pollen.

For about 14 years now, I have avoided dairy products except during school holidays when I eat yogurt or icecream nearly every day. The results are the slow development of a blocked nose until people ask me if I have a cold, a slowly developing loose cough, snoring, and eventually, mucus running down the back of my throat. At that stage I give up and go back to calcium fortified soy products. If I have dairy products during the pollen season, I get hayfever. Because these symptoms develop slowly, I doubt that any would have shown up in the Flinders trial, except the loose cough which was not measured.

Frequent ear infections

Cow's milk and other foods have been associated with frequent ear infections. In Finland, researchers followed up more than 50 children who had been diagnosed with cow's milk allergy under the age of two. They found that even with proper treatment, a diagnosis of milk allergy in infancy was a significant risk for developing recurrent ear infections, usually defined as three episodes in six months or four episodes in 12 months. Children who later developed asthma or hayfever were more likely than controls to have suffered recurrent ear infections and/or glue ear. In Washington, children with recurrent ear infections were evaluated for food allergy and followed an elimination diet for 16 weeks. The diet led to a lessening of symptoms in 85 per cent of children. A challenge with the suspect foods provoked a recurrence of glue ear in 95 per cent.

Sam's father has asthma. Sam was exclusively breastfed until six months, then solids were slowly introduced. He was a happy healthy baby until nine months when he was introduced to cow's milk. Soon after he developed his first ear infection. 'Everything happened at once,' his mother said. 'He had an ear infection, took antibiotics, developed bronchitis and was finally diagnosed with asthma.' He ended up on inhaled corticosteroids and ipratropium. By 14 months, Sam had three more ear infections, each ending in asthma and each needing six weeks of asthma medication.

Antibiotic syrups are often baby's first introduction to high doses of food colours and artificial flavours (p. 83). Experts no longer recommend antibiotics for ear infections. Since pain is the main problem, they recommend treating children for pain. Less than 3 per cent of children with ear infections will go on to develop complications which require antibiotics.

Dairy products as a source of nutrients

Central to the NAC's education campaign about dairy products is the fact that milk is a nutritious food. Cutting out dairy foods can be potentially harmful as dairy foods are the primary source of calcium in the Australian diet and also contribute significant quantities of protein, riboflavin, and Vitamins A and B12. By avoiding dairy products, people with asthma, particularly young children or those with a chronic illness, can risk malnutrition and osteoporosis.

This is an important point, although I feel uncomfortable that the NAC's campaign was organised collaboratively with the Dairy Corporation. A review of osteoporosis by the independent scientists at the Center for Science in the Public Interest in the US includes advice from osteoporosis expert Conrad Johnston at the Indiana University School of Medicine. According to him, as long as you get enough calcium, it doesn't matter whether you get your calcium from a food, a supplement, or the growing number of fortified foods.

Well known Australian nutritionist Rosemary Stanton advises that for those who do not drink milk, calcium is available from soy beverages with absorption about 75% that of dairy milk. Some soy milks have added calcium, Vitamin B12, riboflavin and Vitamin A. These soymilks are considered to be the nutritional equivalent of milk. As well, even in those which contain soy isolate rather than whole beans, you are getting nutrients from the soy beans. Stanton suggests choosing a soy milk which includes Vitamin B12 in the ingredients list.

Asthmatics and bone loss

Osteoporosis is a particularly important issue for asthmatics since certain asthma medications may be associated with bone loss. At first it was thought that bone loss associated with oral steroids could be avoided by using inhaled steroids such as prednisone and cortisone, the most commonly used medications for the long-term treatment of patients with asthma but a study has shown that bone loss is also associated with long-term use of inhaled steroids.

Calcium and bone loss

Like asthma and other diseases of affluence, osteoporosis involving bone loss and hip fractures is associated with the Western lifestyle. Two million Australians are estimated to have the condition, or one in two women and one in three men over the age of 50. Rich countries like Germany and Sweden have 40 times as many hip fractures as poor countries like Thailand. This is despite a calcium intake in poor countries of less than a third of the recommended amount each day.

It has been known for years that certain lifestyle factors are *calcium depleters*:

- phosphates in cola drinks
- sodium—including salt hidden in processed foods
- caffeine in coffee, flavoured milk, cola, energy drinks and icecream
- acid-forming foods like hard cheeses, meats, grains
- smoking
- lack of exercise.

Experts recommend that no woman over 50 should drink more than two cups of coffee a day, or eat processed foods loaded with salt more than three times a week. Teenagers, who are right in the middle of their best bone-building years, should forget soft drinks and 'energy drinks'. Some other *calcium protectors* are:

- exercise
- base-forming foods like fruit and vegetables
- neutralising substances like potassium and sodium bicarbonate.

Professor Maria Fiatarone, a lecturer in the School of Exercise Science at the University of Sydney, considers that the most catastrophic examples of osteoporosis occur in people on long-term doses of drugs like anti-inflammatory steroids. She recommends weight bearing exercise, not calcium supplementation, as the most effective way to build bone and prevent osteoporosis. 'Nobody should be on prednisone without being prescribed a weight-training program,' she says.

Some nutritionists and osteoporosis experts even question the wisdom of recommending extra calcium while eating a typical Western diet. They suggest that the combination of acid-forming foods like cheese, meat and grains which cause bone loss is one of the most important factors in this increase. Base-forming foods like fruit and vegetables are known to protect against bone loss but there may be another way.

In the 1920s, doctors noticed that doses of bicarbonate—a base which neutralises acids—given to kidney patients for bloated stomachs also built sturdier bones. Frequent doses of soda bicarbonate are not a good idea for people with blood pressure problems, but a recent pilot study gave 18 healthy postmenopausal women potassium bicarbonate to neutralise the acid produced by their diets. The results were major, says researcher Dr Anthony Sebastian from the University of California. The women lost *27 per cent less calcium* in their urine than the control group and all the chemical indicators suggested it was because no bone was being broken down. A larger trial is

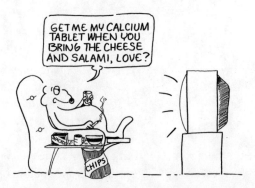

being planned. In the future we may all be taking potassium bicarbonate as well as calcium supplements to protect our bones. In the meantime, we can exercise more and reduce soft drinks, caffeine, cigarettes and processed foods.

The failsafe diet recommended in this book is low in many of the calcium depleters listed above. As well, sodium or potassium bicarbonate has long been recommended as a remedy for food intolerance symptoms (see p. 179).

A couple in their sixties who have been failsafe for four years reported, 'My wife and I recently had our latest bone density tests. We both have had a great increase in bone strength, and we have made no effort to ensure a good calcium intake. My wife's bone strength is 115% of the age-corrected value and has a low risk of fracture. Both of us have bones stronger than we had two years ago!'

9 Medication can be a health hazard

Summary

- The safety of new drugs is not guaranteed. Serious adverse side effects can often appear after the drug has been in use for some years.
- Gifts from pharmaceutical companies may influence doctors to choose drugs by brand rather than effectiveness.
- Patients and doctors may not recognise symptoms which have been caused or worsened by drugs.
- Additives in some drugs can make asthma worse. Avoid sulphites, benzoates and colours whenever possible.
- Some drugs can make asthma worse. In particular, salicylates in many drugs are dangerous for salicylate-sensitive asthmatics.
- Some asthma drugs can make asthma worse.
- You can minimise your risk: avoid unnecessary medications, avoid unnecessary additives in medication, be aware of your sensitivities.

No drug is completely safe. In the US, medical treatments are now the third leading cause of death, after cancer and heart disease. Over a quarter of a million people a year die from the adverse effects of health care. Worldwide, a major contributor to these statistics is the unintended side effects of prescribed medication.

The safety of new drugs is not guaranteed by US Food and Drug Administration (FDA) approval. Within 20 years, one in every five new drugs approved will be withdrawn or be the subject of a black box warning in the physician's reference manual, due to serious side effects. Millions of patients are exposed to potentially unsafe drugs each year.

Pharmaceutical companies also provide gifts, meals, conference travel and accommodation to doctors in the hope that it may remind them to prescribe those companies' products.

The best way to avoid adverse reactions to drugs is to avoid any drugs which are not absolutely essential.

Rules for taking drugs

● Use as few drugs as possible.
● Assume that any new symptom you develop after starting a new drug—including worsening asthma—might be caused by the drug. Patients and doctors may fail to recognise symptoms as the side effects of drugs because they can occur hours, days or longer after starting the drug.

WHAT THE MEDICAL JOURNALS SAY

'[Pharmaceutical company involvement] leads to "nonrational prescribing".'

Wazana A, Is a gift ever just a gift? Physicians and the pharmaceutical industry, *JAMA* 2000;283(3):373–80.

'The safety of new agents cannot be known with certainty until a drug has been on the market for many years.'

Lasser KE, Timing of new black box warnings and withdrawals for prescription medications, *JAMA* 2002 May 1;287(17):2215–20.

- The proper treatment for drug-induced reactions is not a second drug to treat the problem caused by the first drug, but reducing or stopping the first drug.
- Stay with one doctor or pharmacist who knows of all the drugs you are taking, or show each new doctor every medication you take to prevent adverse drug interactions.

Some adverse drug reactions

- exacerbation of asthma
- depression, hallucinations, confusion, delirium, memory loss, impaired thinking, irritability, restless legs and insomnia
- parkinsonism, involuntary movements or spasms of the eyes, face, neck, arms, and legs, stuttering, dizziness on standing, falls, car accidents that result in injury because of sedation or impaired concentration, and sexual dysfunction
- gastrointestinal symptoms: dry mouth, loss of appetite, nausea, vomiting, abdominal pain, bleeding, constipation and diarrhoea
- difficulty urinating or loss of bladder control (incontinence)
- itchy rash, hives
- see also the list of side effects on your consumer medication information (CMI) sheet.

Patients and doctors may not recognise that symptoms have been caused or worsened by drugs. When my son took anti-nausea tablets for a stomach bug in Egypt, I knew that involuntary movements or spasms could be drug induced. But I didn't relate 'involuntary spasms' to his rapid loss of ability to walk, see or breathe. When my aunt was rushed to hospital with life-threatening internal bleeding, neither she nor her doctor related her condition to the arthritis medication she had been taking.

Drugs can be taken by mouth in tablets, capsules or syrups, injected, intravenously through a drip, applied to the skin in a lotion or ointment, inserted rectally as suppositories, inhaled, applied in eye drops or applied to your teeth and gums by your dentist. There have been reports of reactions to drugs with all of these methods. There has even been a life-threatening reaction to artificial colour in an enema (p. 289). Injected additives are likely to cause a stronger reaction.

You should always read the consumer medicine information (CMI) sheet that comes with your medication or look up your drug on the internet. For information on Australian drugs visit www.mydr.com.au, for US drugs, www.my.webMD.com. You also need to check the ingredients listed in the CI (consumer information). Be wary of drugs which warn asthmatics in the CI, or list the following in the PI (prescribing information):

- **Contra**: asthma, aspirin or NSAID sensitive asthma
- **Precaution**: asthma
- **Adverse**: bronchospasm
- **Interact**: any drug you are already taking

Additives in drugs can make asthma worse

There are many reports of life-threatening reactions in asthmatics triggered by additives in drugs. Any additive which can trigger acute asthma attacks in a few can also contribute to bronchial hyperresponsiveness in many more. This is a more subtle reaction which can lead to chronic asthma. It is a particular problem with any drug which you are expected to take long term.

Over the years, sulphites have been removed from many drugs which are used to treat asthma, but not from other drugs which may be given to asthmatics. Other potentially harmful additives such as colours have not been removed. Preservatives are now required to be listed on drug labels, except for the particular class of preservatives called antioxidants (gallates 310–312 and TBHQ, BHA and BHT 319–321). You will find colours not on labels but on the consumer information sheet.

Artificial colours, flavours and preservatives are not failsafe whether in foods or drugs. Avoid them if possible. Flavours used in medications are very strong and more likely to cause reactions than added flavours in foods. The following examples suggest how to find out what is in your drugs and how to avoid potentially harmful active and 'inert' ingredients.

Please note that, as with foods, ingredients in drugs can change at any time. At the time of writing, the following information was correct but may have changed.

Antihistamines

Phenergan (*promethazine hydrochloride*): antihistamine syrup is commonly given to children to treat allergies, for colds and sedation. When I checked, it contained sodium metabisulphite (223), sodium sulphite (221) and sodium benzoate (211), all potential 'asthma additives'. There is also an orange flavour which may affect salicylate-sensitive asthmatics.

The colour in the **Phenergan tablet** is blue opaspray, according to the CMI sheet from manufacturer Aventis Pharma. To find out more information you need to phone the manufacturer or search the Internet. Colours beginning with the prefix 'opa' are tints created for the pharmaceutical industry. Blue opaspray contains titanium dioxide (171, white, failsafe) and indigotine (132, indigo carmine, blue #2). This is what *Additive Code Breaker* has to say about colour 132: 'People with a history of allergy should avoid this colour. May cause nausea, vomiting, high blood pressure and occasionally allergic reactions such as skin rash, itching and breathing problems.'

What you can do: choose a white tablet instead, like Teldane (*terfenadine*) or Claratyne (*loratidine*). No drug is completely safe. An antihistamine named Hismanal was removed from the market several years after receiving black-box warnings for potentially fatal heart problems in certain patients.

Antibiotics

Ceclor (*cefaclor monohydrate*): antibiotic syrup for infections of the respiratory tract including ears, nose, throat, tonsils, chest and lungs is used for babies and children. When I checked, it was coloured pink with artificial colour erythrosine (127, red #3). The information sheet stated 'does not contain tartrazine or any other azo dyes'. This is correct but consumers may think this means the pink colour is harmless. Erythrosine is an artificial coal tar dye. Coal tar dyes have been found to potentially cause adverse effects and erythrosine has been associated with asthma.

What you can do: check with your doctor that an antibiotic is really necessary. The latest medical thinking is that most children will recover from ear infections without the use of antibiotics. Antibiotic use in early childhood is associated with later development of asthma and is now not recommended (see p. 119).

Avoid syrups, suspensions, mixtures and liquid preparations which contain potentially harmful additives. Ask for **white tablets**. Chewable fruit flavours are not OK. If not available, **wash coating off** coloured tablets by rubbing between thumb and forefinger under a running tap. **Capsules**: empty the powdered contents of coloured capsules into a cup and mix with maple syrup, golden syrup, failsafe jam or a spoonful of dairy or soy icecream. If you can't find an alternative, you will have to take the antibiotic and put up with the possibility of consequences.

Cold and flu preparations, cough syrups and lozenges

These medications are for the relief of symptoms only. They are not essential medications. The ingredients lists are a smorgasbord of artificial colours, flavours and preservatives. When I checked, Demazin syrup contained quinoline yellow (104), brilliant blue (133), benzoate preservatives and peach and vanilla flavour. Dimetapp syrup contained allura (129, red #40), brilliant blue (133, blue #1), sodium benzoate and grape flavour. Other medications and throat lozenges were similar. Clear colour-free versions will also contain preservatives and flavours. Demazin Clear contained benzoates and menthol flavour. The CMI sheet warned 'Do not give Demazin Clear to children who have breathing problems and children with asthma . . . unless under the direction of your doctor'. Actifed CC Junior listed asthma as a precaution.

What you can do: Bisolvon (*bromhexine hydrochloride*) white tablets are a useful mucolytic, helping to loosen mucus in both airways and ears. See pp. 212–13 for non-drug cold remedies and failsafe antihistamines above.

Local anaesthetics

There are some accounts of life-threatening reactions to local anaesthetics from dentists, who generally don't expect their patients to die in the chair.

What you can do: ask for an anaesthetic without sulphites or benzoates, for example, plain Xylocaine.

Antacid tablets and powders
The active ingredients such as sodium bicarbonate, calcium carbonate, magnesium carbonate, magnesium sulphate and tartaric acid in antacids are failsafe, and are antidotes for food intolerance symptoms. Avoid syrups and any tablets or powders with colours and flavours including peppermint. Lemon can be OK if it is citric acid.

What you can do: Eno Powder and Sal Vital are failsafe. Or you can make your own, see Antidotes, p. 179.

Some drugs can make asthma worse
Salicylates
Salicylates in drugs have been responsible for some deaths and many life-threatening reactions in asthmatics. You must avoid these during your elimination diet or the diet may not work.

Avoid any drug containing aspirin, salicylic acid, methyl salicylate or similar, menthol, eucalyptus oil, oil of winter-green, mint, peppermint, spearmint, pine oil, camphor or fruit flavours.

Pain relievers, arthritis medication, period pain medication, liniments and pain relievers that you rub on are a common source of salicylates. Always read the ingredients list for every drug.

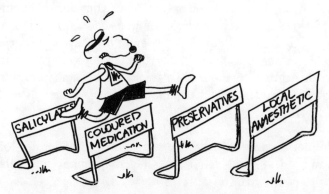

Aspirin

Aspirin (acetylsalicylic acid) is in drugs like: Action Cold and Flu Effervescent, Alka-Seltzer, Asasantin SR, Aspalgin, Aspro Preparations, Astrix, Astrix Bex Powders, Cardiprin 100, Cartia, Codiphen, Codis, Codox, Codral Forte, Disprin, Ecotrin, Morphalgin, Solprin, Spren, Veganin, Vincent's Powders.

Non-steroidal anti-inflammatory drugs (NSAIDs)

These are pain relievers used for pain and inflammatory disorders. They include COX-2 inhibitors and will list 'aspirin or NSAID-sensitive asthma' under precautions in prescribing information. Some examples:

Celecoxib (Celebrex), diclofenac (any medication with that name, also Arthrotec, Diclohexal, Dinac, Fenac, Hexal Diclac, Voltaren), flurbiprofen (Ocufen, Strepfen), ibuprofen (ACT-3, Actiprofen, Brufen, Bugesic, Nurofen, Rafen, Sudafed Congestion & Sinus Pain Relief, Tri-Profen), indomethacin (Arthrexin, Indocid), ketoprofen (Orudis, Oruvail SR), mefenamic acid (Mefic, Ponstan), naproxen (Inza, Naprosyn, Proxen SR), naproxen sodium (Aleve, Anaprox, Crysanal, Naprogesic, Nurolasts), piroxicam (any medication with that name, also Candyl, Feldene, Mobilis, Pirohexal-D, Rosig), Rofecoxib (Vioxx).

What you can do: if possible, use paracetamol (called acetaminophen in the US) or codeine white tablets instead. After some highly-publicised deaths, the US FDA warned that paracetamol can cause liver damage and death at doses not much higher than those recommended as 'safe'. Never exceed recommended doses of this or any other drug. For children, it is necessary to calculate dose per kilogram of body weight, crush tablet and see serving suggestions on p. 84.

Absorption through skin: avoid preparations you rub or spray on your skin which contain salicylic acid, methyl or other salicylates and NSAIDS.

Liniments, pain relieving rubs

Avoid salicylates, NSAIDs, menthol and camphor in preparations such as: Biosal arthritis cream, Deep Heat, Dencorub,

---

FROM THE MEDICAL JOURNALS

Methyl salicylate (oil of wintergreen) is widely available in many over–the–counter liniments, ointments, lotions or medicated oils for the relief of musculoskeletal aches and pains . . . Methyl salicylate in topical analgesic preparations may cause irritant or allergic contact dermatitis and anaphylactic reactions.

Chan TY, Potential dangers from topical preparations containing methyl salicylate, *Hum Exp Toxicol* 1996 Sep;15(9):747–50.

Hexal Diclac Anti-inflammatory Gel (diclofenac), Ice Gel, Linsal, Metsal Analgesic Gel and liniment, Movelat Sportz, Orudis Gel, Radian-B, Rubesal, Voltaren Eulgel, Zam-Buk herbal balm.

Teething gel and mouth pain

Avoid salicylates in preparations such as: Bonjela, Ora-sed Jel, SM-33 Gel.

Wart and corn removers

Avoid salicylic acid in preparations such as Clear Away Wart Remover System, Cornkil, Dermatech Wart Treatment, Duofilm, Posalfilin. Choose alternatives.

Acne treatments and skin cleansers

Avoid salicylic acid in preparations such as Clearasil Medicated Foam and Wipes, Curaderm. Choose alternatives.

Medicated shampoos, prickly heat and skin treatments

For example, Egozite Cradle Cap Lotion, Foltene Research Anti-Dandruff Shampoo, Goanna Analgesic Ice, Ionil, Mycoderm, Psor-Asist, Sebitar, SOOV Prickly Heat Powder, Sunspot Cream, Superfade Cream.

Vicks Vaporub

Used as a rub or inhalant for nasal congestion. When I checked, this treatment contained menthol, camphor, thymol, eucalytus oil, turpentine oil, nutmeg oil and cedarwood oil. It can cause real problems for people who are sensitive to salicylates. See p. 213 for alternatives.

Salicylates in flavours, toothpastes and herbal remedies
Fruit and mint flavours in drugs and toothpaste are very high in salicylates. All fresh herbs contain salicylates except parsley. Dried herbs and extracts contain even more salicylates because they are concentrated, so remedies and supplements which contain herbs or bioflavonoids are not failsafe. Herbal tooth-paste flavoured with fennel or other herbs is not a low salicylate substitute for mint-flavouring. Even aloe vera strips on razors can cause reactions in the salicylate-sensitive.

Other drugs associated with asthma
Beta-blockers
Beta-blockers such as Inderal (propranolol) used to treat high blood pressure, cardiac disorders and migraine may affect asthmatics. Prescribing information will list bronchospasm and allergic disorders as a 'contra' or reason not to take these drugs.

Eye drops used to treat glaucoma
Beta blockers can also be used in eye drops to treat glaucoma. These include Cosopt, Tenopt, Timoptol and Timpilo (timolol). Glaucoma preparations containing carbachol or pilocarpine can have the same effects. If you have to use them, apply pressure to the inside corner of the eye immediately after application.

Cholinesterase inhibitors
Muscle relaxants such as Mestinon (pyridostygmine) have been associated with bronchial asthma.

Sedatives
Sedatives are not recommended during an acute asthma attack as most cause reduced respiratory drive.

When a young woman was discovered dead at home, an

autopsy found she had died of an asthma attack following an overdose of a commonly used anti-depressant. Authorities were unsure whether the drug had contributed to the attack or prevented her from being aware of the asthma until too late.

Some asthma drugs can make asthma worse

No drug suits everyone. In Japan, a 39-year-old man with adult onset asthma nearly died when he used his daughter's sodium cromoglycate nebuliser because his own puffer was not enough. Sodium cromoglycate is considered to be one of the safest asthma medications on the market but there are always exceptions. Montelukast was launched as a revolutionary new asthma treatment, 'a pill a day keeps asthma at bay', however increasing reports may link montelukast and other leukotriene inhibitors with Churg-Strauss Syndrome, a severe form of asthma (see p. 109).

It is very important to tell your doctor if your medication is not working. Many patients suffer and a significant number die or are permanently disabled before a 'bad' drug will be withdrawn.

Puffers without puff

In 2000, a giant pharmaceutical company in the USA issued a recall for 59 million asthma inhalers, based on the possibility that they might not contain any active ingredient. It is difficult

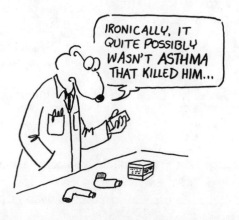

for patients, their families, or doctors to believe that an asthma inhaler could fail to contain the asthma drug. You can read more at http://www.citizen.org/publications/release.cfm?ID=7049 and http://www.ClassActionAmerica.com/cases/case.asp?cid=989&categoryID=5.

Preservatives in drugs

The adverse effects of sulphites in both foods and drugs are well known. Benzalkonium chloride (BAC), a preservative used only in drugs, has been found to be potentially harmful to asthmatics. Most Western countries have removed these additives from most asthma drugs except for the US. When the US FDA proposed that all bronchodilator solutions should be made sterile and pre-servative-free, they were opposed by at least one drug manufac-turer. Currently only about half the available bronchodilator solutions are preservative-free. Some hospitals choose sulphite-preserved medications because they are cheaper.

When I checked, adrenaline inhalers, now unavailable in the UK and Australia, contained sulphite preservatives. Isopre-naline, now available only in injections in Australia, still con-tained sodium bisulphite.

Metered dose aerosol bronchodilators such as Ventolin inhalers do not contain sulphites. Despite pleas from numerous doctors in

---

FROM THE MEDICAL JOURNALS

'Although primary exposure in children is through foods, serious reactions have also occurred after oral, inhalational, parenteral and ophthalmic administration of sulfite–containing drugs.'

American Academy of Pediatrics, 'Inactive' ingredients in pharmaceutical products, *Pediatrics* 1997; 99(2):268–78.

'Despite an abundance of asthmatic and anaphylaxis–like reac-tions associated with their use, sulfite containing solutions . . . continue to be available and are used by a few institutions to save money . . .'

Asmus MJ and others, Bronchoconstrictor additives in bronchodilator solutions, *J Allergy Clin Immunol* 1999;104:S53–60.

medical journals to remove potentially harmful preservatives from asthma drugs there are still sulphite and BAC-preserved asthma treatments on the market and used in hospitals in the US.

What can be done: 'We recommend that the United States follow the practice of most Western countries and withdraw bronchodilator nebuliser solutions that contain preservatives', concluded a New Zealand research team. There is an alternative. Preservative-free solutions can be prepared under sterile conditions and made available in unit-dose vials.

In Australia, adrenaline injections recommended for use with 'acute allergic reactions with airways obstruction' still contain sodium bisulphite, while listing sulfite content as a precaution. If you know you are sensitive to sulphites, wear a medical alert bracelet saying so.

In the US, epinephrine (adrenaline) inhalers are still available over the counter. These inhalers are considered to be safe and effective when used occasionally for mild, intermittent asthma but surveys suggest that 20 per cent of users are likely to use their inhalers more than recommended. Overuse of these products can cause severe adverse reactions, including death. These inhalers may contain sulphites.

Steroids
Methylprednisolone and other steroids are standard in the management of acute asthma attacks. There are occasional reports of adverse reactions including bronchospasm, respiratory arrest and anaphylaxis.

Be alarmed—be very alarmed
CMI sheets are reassuring. 'Do not be alarmed by this list of possible side effects', they say. 'You may not experience any of them'. Maybe not, but in the US there are over 100,000 deaths per year from the side effects of drugs. There are many more near deaths and severe reactions, including some resulting in permanent disability. Patients with asthma are among the most vulnerable. Patients and doctors may not recognise that symptoms have been caused or worsened by drugs.

What you can do: avoid asthma medications which contain preservatives, especially sulphites, benzoates and benzalkonium chloride. Avoid hospitals if possible by keeping your asthma under control. Do your elimination diet with challenges so you know whether your asthma is sensitive to sulphites, benzoates, colours and salicylates used in drugs. Wear a medical alert bracelet with this information.

Hospital food can be a health hazard

In hospital, you are at risk from food additives and salicylates in both drugs and food. Remember the Danish hospital study on p. 5? During the trial, three patients eating hospital food suffered severe asthmatic attacks including one respiratory and cardiac arrest compared to none on the 'grey glop' diet.

What you can do: request the Royal Prince Alfred Hospital elimination diet. Hospital dietitians unfamiliar with this diet can obtain information from RPAH (see p. 300).

10 A call to arms

Summary
- The time has come for us to reduce the causes of asthma, instead of throwing more drugs and money at its management.
- The effects of food additives have been seriously underestimated.
- The use of additives known to be potentially harmful should be banned or minimised.
- Information about any amount of any additive in foods should be clearly labelled and available at point of sale.
- Change what you eat and change the world. *Refuse to buy* additive-laden foods, sign the tartrazine petition (on p. 301) and spread the word.

The rate of asthma is increasing almost all over the world and Australia is one of the worst affected countries. A survey in 1997 found almost four children in 10 had been diagnosed with asthma and nearly one in two had taken medication for asthma. The rate of wheeze has been increasing by 1.5 per cent a year for 15 years. Every year about 500 Australians die of asthma.

The National Asthma Council advises we should take preventive medication; however, the prevalence of asthma is still rising. The costs to our community are also dramatic: approximately $700 million a year.

The time has come for us to prevent asthma, instead of throwing more drugs and money at its management. My experience, backed by medical studies, suggests that about half of asthmatic adults and two-thirds of asthmatic children can be helped by avoiding certain food chemicals.

You can improve your or your child's asthma through changing what you eat. As an individual you can also help to reduce the worldwide burden of asthma.

Step 1: Change what you eat
For most asthmatics, avoiding sulphites will make a big difference, but this is easier said than done. See pp. 187–93 for detailed

---

WHAT THE RESEARCHERS SAY

'It is now clear that sulphites are not safe preservatives . . . The food industry, including beer and wine manufacturers, and the pharmaceutical industry, should consider using alternatives.'
Yang WH and Purchase ECR, Adverse reactions to sulphites, *Can Med Assoc J* 1985; 133:865–67.

'The obvious public–health response would be to remove the irritants, if possible, from the foods that children eat . . . the FDA should consider banning the use of synthetic dyes in foods widely consumed by children because dyes adversely affect some children and do not offer any essential benefits.'
Jacobson FJ and Schardt D, 1999, Diet, ADHD and behaviour: a quarter–century review, *Centre for Science in the Public Interest.*

instructions. I recommend a trial of the failsafe diet, partly to find out exactly which food chemicals affect you, and partly as a way of learning exactly what is in our foods. You will be surprised.

Step 2: Change the world

This is what we need to campaign for:

- Sulphites banned in all foods except wine. There are alternatives. The use of sulphites should be minimised in wine.
- All potentially harmful colours banned. This includes all azo dyes, coal tar dyes, annatto and cochineal. They serve no useful purpose and there are alternatives.
- *Every* ingredient should be listed on food labels. No 5 per cent labelling loophole (see box on p. 203).
- Use of the 50 harmful additives (p. 231) should be minimised.
- When MSG or its equivalent (for example, in HVP or HPP) is present *in any amount* in a product, the quantity should be listed on the label.
- Accurate information about every ingredient in every food should be available at point of sale, including restaurants.
- A national government-funded, industry-independent organisation should collect and monitor reports of adverse reactions to drugs and food additives.
- The effect of genetic engineering on salicylate levels in foods should be monitored.

How can we achieve this?

The food industry will resist and say there is no evidence that additives may cause harm. But the time for debate is over. Studies and researchers have shown that additives can harm.

Regulators around the world supposedly protect consumer rights and standards. However, they don't seem to have much power at all when it comes to influential food industry lobby groups.

The way to change regulations about food is to create a public outcry. This was shown to be effective more than 100 years ago when a public outcry about the use of poisonous lead salts as food colours led to their ban.

There are alternatives

Food technologists say there are safe and effective alternatives to artificial food colours and sulphites in all foods except wine.

There is a precedent

A similar change to the one I am proposing occurred in 1989 in New Zealand. At that time New Zealand was in the grip of a terrible epidemic of asthma deaths. When researchers suggested the cause may be a particular type of asthma medication, the department of health allowed 'an experiment in prevention' by restricting availabilty of the drug.

Within six months, the asthma death rate had dropped dramatically and within 12 months it had halved and has remained at the lower level. Academics are still debating whether the drug caused the deaths, but at the end of the day lives have been saved. We are concerned here not only with saving lives, but also reducing the incidence of asthma.

It's up to us

People will not change what they eat unless they are desperate. Parents of asthmatic children are not necessarily desperate enough. As one mother said, 'She's no trouble at all when she's got asthma. She just sits there and tries to breathe.'

Nothing will happen to make our food safer unless consumers like you and me make enough noise. Here are some simple things you can do:

- **First: sign the petitions**: see p. 301.
- **Second: refuse to buy**: money talks. If enough consumers refuse to buy food products and medications containing sulphites and other harmful additives, the food industry will change their tune overnight. You will be protecting your own health and that of asthmatics all over the world at the same time.
- **Third: contact the media**: tell your story, or that of your child, or any asthmatic you know of who has improved as a result of avoiding these additives to your favourite media. You could choose a magazine which publishes reader's

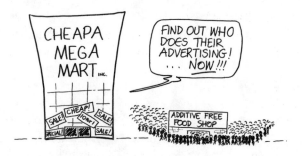

opinions and stories; a letter to the editor of your local or national newspaper; or an email bulletin board. There's also the websites of the big current affairs programs—they always have an invitation such as 'got a story for us?'. Tell them your story or give them some feedback about any features they have done on asthma and what you think they should do. You could also contact your local Asthma Foundation (p. 299) asking them to support a ban on sulphites and harmful colours.

Thank you for your help!

part two

Asthma Prevention and Management

11 Asthma can be fatal

Summary
- No-one ever thinks they are going to die from asthma.
- There are about 500 asthma deaths per year in Australia. Many of them are preventable.
- Many people with asthma believe the severity of their asthma is not as bad as it really is and that their management of it is better than it actually is.
- Medications for asthma have different purposes. Relievers are often overused, preventers are often underused.
- The potential side effects of asthma medication can be minimised.
- Peak flow meters, puffers, spacers and other devices assist in the effective management of asthma.
- Know the warning signs of an asthma attack and have an asthma action plan.

Asthma can be fatal but people never think they are going to die from an asthma attack. They often believe their asthma is not as bad as it really is and that their management is better than it actually is. You don't have to have severe asthma to die. Studies of asthma deaths and near deaths show that asthmatics and their relatives are likely to call for help too late.

A child with severe asthma will be very quiet. Often there is no wheeze. They will be struggling to breathe and unable to talk much. They may sit up to help the lungs inflate. All the muscles of the neck, back, chest and abdomen are used. You can see a hollow at the base of the throat and the outline of the ribs as the breath is sucked in. Usually they have a blue tinge around the lips. The hard work needed to drag more air into the lungs makes them very tired. If this happens for too long, they become too exhausted to continue breathing and there is a danger of respiratory arrest.

What *is* asthma?

Asthma is a transient and reversible narrowing of the airways. Symptoms of asthma can include any or all of the following:
- a dry hacking cough which can become a moist, mucus producing cough
- tightness in the chest
- shortness of breath
- wheezing.

Severity of asthma in Australian children

About three quarters of all children with asthma will have isolated episodes of asthma that last from a few days to two weeks, usually more than two months apart. The episodes are normally triggered by an upper respiratory tract infection or exposure to an allergen. There are no symptoms between episodes. Although most episodes are mild, this group accounts for up to 60 per cent of hospital admissions for asthma. About 20 per cent of children with asthma have more frequent episodes with symptoms such as exercise-induced asthma between episodes. Five to 10 per cent of asthmatic children have persistent asthma with acute episodes plus symptoms on most days in between.

About 60 per cent of adults with asthma will have symptoms less than once a week, with occasional symptoms after triggers such as exercise.

About 25 per cent of asthmatic adults have frequent episodes of wheezing up to three times a week and a further 10 per cent have symptoms every day. They avoid sports and exercise, and experience sleep disturbance at least once a week.

Of adults with severe asthma, five per cent will be chronically ill with frequent wheezing during the day, serious sleep disturbance and limited lifestyle. Half will be admitted to hospital at some time. For about 1 per cent of all asthmatic adults, asthma is an incapacitating illness. They experience disabling symptoms every day, and multiple hospital admissions.

Is your asthma well managed?

You will know your asthma is poorly managed if you have the following signs:

- Needing a blue reliever puffer (for example, salbutamol, Ventolin) more than three times a week.
- Waking at night because of asthma.
- Missing work or school because of asthma.
- Almost daily asthma symptoms.

Most people don't like the idea of taking medication all the time whether they need it or not. Unfortunately, with asthma, this can be the best way to relieve symptoms and avoid side effects.

How bad is your asthma?

A quick gauge as to the severity of asthma is how much you can talk:

- Can talk whole sentences—mild asthma
- Can talk only in phrases—moderate asthma
- Can manage only single words, like your name, or 'I'm asthmatic'—severe asthma.

Peak flow meters

A more sophisticated way of monitoring asthma is by using a peak flow meter which measures lung capacity. You can assess how bad your asthma is and whether an attack is imminent. Chronic asthmatics can take daily readings while mild asthmatics can check when needed. Peak flow meters can also measure the effectiveness of medication, improvements in lung capacity, and the effects of food chemicals while on the elimination diet.

Peak flow readings vary depending on age, height and gender. It is useful to know:

- your best peak flow level
- the level at which you need to increase medication
- the level at which you need urgent medical attention.

What's your peak flow reading?

Stand up—put the marker on zero or start—hold the peak flow meter level—take a deep breath—put the peak flow meter in your mouth and close your lips around it tightly—blow out as hard and fast as possible—check the number—take the best reading of three.

Peak flow meter problems

You can chart your readings on a graph. This can be used to fine-tune your medication—provided the readings are accurate.

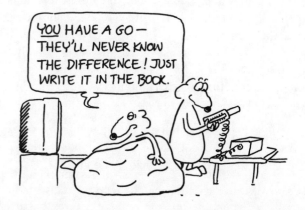

In a Dutch study, children were asked to chart their readings using an electronic peak flow meter which kept a record of all readings, although the participants didn't know that. Their handwritten charts were found to be less than 50 per cent accurate. Many had filled in the gaps with made-up readings.

Where to buy
The cheapest place to buy a peak flow meter is from your local Asthma Foundation. See contact details p. 299, however they are also available from pharmacies.

Side effects of asthma versus medication
All drugs have potential side effects and some are worse than others. The very young, females and the very old are the most vulnerable to side effects. The higher the dose or the longer you take the drug, the more likely you are to be affected but if you don't take the drug, then your unmanaged asthma could result in death. It can also cause abnormal lung function. Some parents worry about asthma medication stunting their child's growth but unmanaged asthma can do that too. The best way to avoid the possible side effects of drugs is to work closely with your doctor to get the best lung function and symptom control with the minimum of side effects.

If you want to avoid asthma medication, you can do the Failsafe diet and, if necessary, breathing techniques, see Chapter 16. But until you improve, you need to continue with your medication. Remember Liz from Chapter 3? Liz's formerly frequent asthma attacks were provoked by sulphites in foods. It took her 20 years of asthma, medication and frequent hospitalisation to find out that sulphites were her problem. She is now attack-free but still at risk:

> Asthma is always with me. Even though I am aware of what I can and can't eat, there is always the chance I could make a mistake, and it could be deadly.

It is impossible to guarantee that the food we eat is sulphite free, especially in restaurants and on social occasions, but also when sulphites are sometimes added illegally to fresh food. *Do not* give up your asthma medication until the other methods are effective. *Consult* your doctor before reducing medication. Some medications must be reduced gradually. You always need to *carry your blue puffer* in case of mistakes.

Medication for asthma

Asthma drugs fall into three categories: relievers (blue puffers), symptom controllers (green puffers) and preventers (brown puffers). You can find information about your asthma drugs, including possible side effects, on the Consumer Medication Information (CMI) in the pack, or on www.mydr.com.au.

Relievers (blue puffers)

Short-acting beta-agonists: salbutamol (e.g. Ventolin, Airomir, Asmol, Epaq) and terbutaline (e.g. Bricanyl turbuhaler).

These are the most widely used drugs for quick relief of asthma. Called bronchodilators because they open up the airways, they work almost immediately and last up to four hours. They are taken on an 'as needed' basis and are extremely effective when used in moderation, but overuse may reduce their effectiveness. Save these guys for when you *really* need them. If you are using a puffer more than three or four times a week, you need to be taking preventive medication.

Possible side effects include: headache, nausea, shaky or tense feeling, 'warm' feeling, fast or irregular heart beat, pounding heart beat. According to the NAC, oral versions—syrup or tablets—should be discouraged because they can take up to an hour to start working and 'the incidence of behavioural side-effects and sleep disturbance is reasonably high'.

Some studies have suggested a rebound effect of these medications. This means that after regular use, stopping the medication may cause an increase in bronchial hyperresponsiveness (BHR) which takes a number of days to return to the original pre-medication level. The rebound effect could account for why some people have difficulty getting off medication even when their asthma is controlled by diet. Breathing techniques (see Chapter 16) may help with this.

Theophylline: (e.g. Neulin).

The use of this drug has decreased because of possible side effects. Long-acting beta-agonists are safer. Theophylline is most likely to be used by people with severe persistent asthma who require multiple drugs to control their symptoms.

Possible side effects: nausea, vomiting, loss of appetite, headaches, sleep disturbance, restlessness, anxiety, irritability, tremor and others. Avoid long-term high doses if possible.

Atropines: ipratropium bromide (e.g. Aproven, Atrovent).

Ipratropium bromide is a mild drug with mild possible side effects. It can take up to an hour to work, so carry a blue puffer as well for acute asthma. Ipratropium bromide is most likely to be used for chronic obstructive pulmonary disease, or initial management of moderate to severe acute asthma in children.

Possible side effects: dry throat and mouth, headache, nausea and more.

Symptom controllers (green puffers)

Long-acting beta-agonists: salmeterol (e.g. Serevent) and eformoterol (e.g. Foradile capsules for inhalation, Oxis).

These are long-acting relievers which last at least 12 hours. They're for people who can't get on top of their symptoms, especially at night.

Possible problems: these drugs can take a while to work. They shouldn't be used when you need fast relief. Always carry a blue puffer as well.

Long-acting beta-agonists protect against exercise and allergens. Protection against exercise-induced asthma begins 30 minutes after inhalation, peaks at two hours, and lasts for up to 12 hours according to some studies, although one study suggests that the protection may be as short as four hours in some patients. If taken daily, they can become less effective in preventing exercise asthma and blocking allergen-induced bronchoconstriction. There are suggestions that the protective effect of these drugs may wear off with regular use.

Possible side effects: similar to those of the short-acting beta agonists—shaking or muscle tremor, headaches and palpitations. Occasional coughing as an immediate reaction to the propellant in metered dose inhalers.

Preventers (brown puffers)

Inhaled corticosteroids: beclomethasone dipropionate (e.g. Qvar), budesonide (e.g. Pulmicort), fluticasone propionate (e.g. Flixotide).

Inhaled corticosteroids are the main preventive therapy for adults and children with moderate to severe persistent asthma. They reduce inflammation and swelling, and cut down the amount of mucus. The idea is to keep taking them even when you are well because when you are exposed to a trigger they will prevent an attack.

Possible problems: potential side effects can be the big problem with corticosteroids. The aim is to keep the dose as low as possible. More is not always better. Inhaled drugs have less possible side effects than those taken by mouth as tablets or syrup. For this reason, oral steroids such as prednisolone are only used as short-term therapy when strictly necessary.

Possible side effects—short term: common local possible side effects include oral thrush and hoarseness. With inhalers these can be reduced by using a valved spacer and oral hygiene after each dose (rinse, gargle and spit). If coughing is a problem with the use of an inhaler, use a spacer or automatic breath-activated device. Possible behavioural side effects include anxiety, aggression and hyperactivity in children.

Possible side effects of long term oral steroids: weight gain, fluid retention, bruising, damaged or thinning skin, stretch marks, skin rash, redness of the face and neck, puffy or round moon-face, bone loss, stomach irritation, peptic ulcers, depression, cataracts, exacerbation of diabetes and high blood pressure, reduced immunity to infections, and glaucoma. The risk of potential side effects is dose-related. Some people are more sensitive than others. For more details, see www.national jewish.org/medfacts/corticosteroids.html.

Growth suppression in children is a possible side effect, but poorly controlled asthma can cause that too. Experts caution

---

WHAT THE PATIENTS SAY

'The side effects which bothered me were headaches, palpitations, the shakes and inability to sleep from the bronchodilators, especially when on the nebuliser or on higher doses of the puffer during an attack.'

---

that nebulised corticosteroids should only be used in infants and young children where the alternative would be an extended course of oral corticosteroids.

The older corticosteroid inhalers which contained CFC (Becloforte, Becotide and Respocort) were withdrawn in 2002.

A new class of preventive drugs for asthma—Leukotriene receptor antagonists: montelukast sodium (e.g. Singulair) and zafirlukast (e.g. Accolate, no longer recommended).

Leukotriene antagonists are a new class of drug recommended particularly for exercise-induced or salicylate-sensitive asthma. Any new drug can be potentially dangerous because possible side effects may not become apparent until the drug has been on the market for a few years. Accolate was approved in 1996. By 2000, there were some reports of liver damage after treatment with zafirlukast. In the medical journal *Annals of Internal Medicine*, doctors warned that patients receiving zafirlukast may develop severe liver injury and should be observed for signs and symptoms of hepatitis, which can include nausea, itching, jaundice and fatigue.

At its Australian release in 1999, montelukast was hailed as 'a pill a day that could keep asthma at bay', the first revolutionary new treatment for asthma in 20 years and a way of avoiding the possible side effects of corticosteroids. Results were said to be so remarkable that many asthmatics would feel as if they no longer had asthma. Montelukast has greatly improved the quality of life for some people with asthma but not others. It is usually used to reduce the large doses of steroids often required by people with moderate to severe asthma to keep their asthma under control.

At first, possible side effects were thought to be temporary headaches and flushing. Within months there were some reports of associated Churg-Strauss Syndrome (CSS), a condition involving worsening asthma, eosinophilia (an increase in white blood cells associated with allergies), vasculitis (skin rashes, arthritis, bruising), cardiac complications, and/or neuropathy (weakness or numbness in the limbs). One of the first cases was a 26-year-old man with a three year history of asthma. After approximately four months of treatment with montelukast the patient developed headache, malaise, muscular aches, nasal congestion and mild fever. Seven days later he developed breathlessness and was admitted to hospital. He improved as soon as montelukast was withdrawn. At first, doctors assumed these patients had pre-existing CSS masked by previous corticosteroid treatment but Norwegian doctors reported the condition in a 20-year-old girl who had never been treated with steroids.

Some possible side effects Mild: headache, stomach pain, nausea, vomiting, diarrhoea, drowsiness, difficulty sleeping, irritability, restlessness, hallucinations (seeing, feeling or hearing things that are not there), muscle aches or muscle cramps and fluid retention. *Serious*: skin rash or itchiness, increased tendency to bleed and bruising.

Inhaled non-steroidal anti-inflammatories: sodium cromoglycate (e.g. Intal) and nedocromil sodium (e.g. Tilade).

These are considered to be the safest of all the asthma drugs. Sodium cromoglycate can be used as first preventive therapy for children with frequent episodic asthma. It is also effective in adults with mild asthma. It inhibits exercise-induced asthma in adults and children if used immediately before exercise and may be useful if used before allergen exposure in susceptible individuals. Benefits are usually obvious within one to two weeks but a four-week trial is recommended before considering other treatments.

Possible side effects: sneezing, coughing (rare); bronchospasm.

Nedocromil sodium: (e.g. Tilade).

This drug is chemically different from drugs like Intal and the corticosteroids. It protects against allergens and exercise for longer, and prevents metabisulfite-induced narrowing of the airways. It is also useful for seasonal allergic asthma. Asthmatic cough may reduce within two to three days of starting medication.

Possible problems: Not all asthmatics respond to this drug. Some people complain about the distinctive taste.

Possible side effects: headache, nausea, minor throat irritation, cough and bronchospasm.

Combination Medications: fluticasone and salmeterol (e.g. Seretide).

Combination medications are a way of reducing the potential adverse effects of high doses of inhaled corticosteroids. Possible side effects are no different when taking the drugs together or separately.

How to take medication: puffers

Medications can be taken though pressurised inhalers (puffers), breath-activated inhalers, nebulisers, as tablets or as a syrup. Puffers provide faster benefits and fewer side effects than the same medication taken by mouth.

Puffer problems: puffers require good coordination. Up to half of all asthma patients fail to use their inhalers correctly. There's no point in taking medication if it doesn't reach your lungs. Check your technique. The use of autohalers and spacers, see below, can improve drug delivery.

To use a puffer: take the cap off and shake puffer a few times, holding upright—take a breath and breathe out to clear the lungs—tilt the head back a bit—close lips tightly around the mouthpiece—place your finger on the top of the puffer and press down hard breathing in *at the same time*—hold breath to the count of 4 to let the medication work—repeat if needed.

Alternatives to puffers which do not require coordination including a breath-activated inhaler (Autohaler) or a dry

---

WARNING: BLOCKAGES IN CFC–FREE INHALERS
CFC–free inhalers are replacing the old CFC–containing inhalers.
The new CFC–free propellant protects the ozone layer but is
stickier than the original and can build up to cause a blockage.
You must wash your inhaler regularly in warm water. See instruc-
tions in the pack.

---

powder inhaler (Turbuhaler, Rotahaler, Accuhaler or Spinhaler).
For very young children a small volume spacer with an attached
face mask can be used.

How to take medication: spacers

When you use a puffer, only about 10 per cent of the medication actually reaches the lungs. This can be increased by the
use of small volume spacers which deliver 20 per cent more
medication to the lungs. You can buy a plastic spacer or
make one yourself by putting a hole in the bottom of a soft-
drink bottle.

To use a spacer: shake—fit inhaler to spacer—activate
inhaler—breathe in and out of spacer four times.

Spacers have largely replaced the use of nebulisers because
they are just as effective and much cheaper.

Spacer problems: compared to inhalers, spacers are big,
bulky and less convenient to carry around. If caught in a situation where a puffer isn't enough, you can improvise a spacer out
of a polystyrene cup or the cardboard middle of a toilet roll.
Helpers at the scene of an asthma attack in a cinema have been

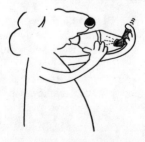

known to run into toilets looking for cardboard tubes. See asthma first aid, p. 114.

AN ASTHMATIC TELLS
'The Asthma Foundation is the best place to buy spacers. They are not as flash as the ones from pharmacies but they are cheaper and more useful. There's a small volume spacer you can put your puffer inside and carry in your handbag or schoolbag.'

Other drugs used to treat asthma

Antibiotics are not a treatment for asthma. When mucus and a productive cough accompany asthma, they do not indicate infection unless there are other symptoms. Antibiotics are only for infections. It is best to use antibiotics only when necessary. Antibiotic use in babies may increase their chance of getting asthma (see p. 119). Antibiotics may contain colours and preservatives associated with asthma (see p. 83).

Antihistamines: doctors used to think that antihistamines would cause mucus secretions in the airway to become drier and thicker and therefore harder to remove. They know now that this does not happen. Antihistamines may be used to treat associated nasal and other allergy symptoms. Be careful: some antihistamines contain preservatives or colours (see p. 83).

Sedatives are not a good idea during an acute attack of asthma as most sedatives reduce the drive to breathe. Agitation during an attack can be due to lack of oxygen. This can be treated with bronchodilators and oxygen.

ALWAYS CARRY A BLUE PUFFER
A woman developed asthma after a sunset champagne picnic in a nature reserve. Unable to walk, she waited in the dark while her husband ran to the car, drove to the nearest farmhouse for an asthma puffer, and ran back. The woman, a health professional, commented later, 'I felt so embarrassed. I tell my patients to carry their puffers and there I was without mine.'

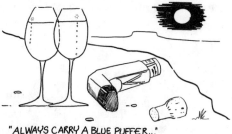

"ALWAYS CARRY A BLUE PUFFER..."

The Australian six-step asthma management plan

Australian deaths caused by asthma rose steadily from 1978 and peaked in 1989 at 964 deaths. Up to 60 per cent of deaths were considered to be avoidable and the death rates were higher in Australia than most other countries. In that year, the Thoracic Society of Australia and New Zealand published management guidelines for asthma care consisting of a six-step plan, the first treatment guidelines in the world.

Their main recommendation is that all people who experience asthma symptoms more than a few times a week should use preventive medication and have an action plan. This recommendation has been adopted as the basis of educational activities conducted by the National Asthma Campaign, now Council (NAC), since 1990. The NAC estimates that 30–40 per cent of asthmatics who need preventive medication are not taking it.

THE SIX STEPS OF THE MANAGEMENT PLAN
1. Know how severe your asthma is.
2. Achieve your best lung function—ideally, no symptoms and best possible peak flow reading.
3. Find out what your trigger factors are and avoid them (pp. 156–211).
4. Maintain your best lung function with optimal medication—preventer medication and reliever medication as needed.
5. Know your action plan—develop this with your doctor so you know how to manage your asthma.
6. Follow your action plan and review it regularly with your doctor.

These are the warning signs of an asthma attack:
- wheezing more often
- persistent dry cough
- increasing breathlessness
- decreasing peak flow readings
- using your puffer more but it doesn't help as much as usual

Your Asthma Action Plan, developed with your doctor, is based on your peak flow readings. It will tell you when to take more medication and when you need to go to hospital. Remember, most asthma deaths result from help not being called soon enough because asthmatics or their carers failed to recognise the severity of their symptoms.

The NAC's campaign for asthmatics to take medication has been highly successful at reducing the asthma death rate by more than half. However, more people continue to get asthma—and more severe asthma.

You can take medication, you can do an elimination diet, you can do breathing lessons or you can do all three. Any way you look at it, doing nothing is the worst thing you can do. Take asthma seriously.

How to save a life—asthma first aid

You are with someone who has an asthma attack. What are you going to do? First aid is based on the **ASTHMA** plan.

Assess	**Mild**
	Moderate
	Severe
Sit	**Upright**
	Stay calm and reassure
Treat	**4 separate puffs of blue/grey Reliever puffer with spacer if available**
	Repeat in 4 minutes if no improvement

Help   **Call ambulance if no improvement or if in doubt**

Monitor   **Observe person**
                Repeat medication if required

All OK?   **If symptoms re-occur repeat emergency procedure**
                If recovered can resume activity

EMERGENCY PROCEDURE FOR ASTHMA RELIEVER WITH SPACER
Place mouthpiece of spacer into mouth (five years and over) or mask of spacer over nose and mouth (under five years).

One puff—4 breaths in and out through spacer
One puff—4 breaths in and out through spacer   } total of
One puff—4 breaths in and out through spacer   } 4 puffs
One puff—4 breaths in and out through spacer

Spacers make asthma medication more effective. With a puffer, only 10% of the medication gets into the lungs. Spacers will allow another 20% into the lungs and get better results. An emergency spacer can be made by punching a hole in the bottom of a polystyrene cup or a soft drink bottle, if you have the tools. Or you can use the cardboard middle of a toilet roll.

COULD YOU DO IT?
Nurse Naomi Rosenberg was managing a backpackers' lodge when a guest had a severe asthma attack. Naomi sat the woman up and administered asthma first aid. The woman drifted in and out of consciousness, throwing up each time she jerked back into consciousness. While waiting for an ambulance, Naomi talked to keep her alert and conscious, and kept her airways clear of vomit. 'It was the hardest thing I've ever done,' recalled Naomi, who won an award—and a job—for her efforts.

12 Asthma in babies and children

Summary
- Some natural foods may help to prevent asthma; some features of the Western lifestyle—bottle feeding, antibiotics, pasteurisation, the wrong kinds of fats in our diet—may contribute to asthma.
- Breastmilk can encourage growth of good bacteria in the gut.
- Antimicrobials like antibiotics and food preservatives which can kill both harmful bacteria and good bacteria are best avoided.
- Probiotics are the opposite of antibiotics. They are good bacteria in fermented milk products like yoghurt. A recently discovered probiotic called Lactobacillus GG appears to be particularly effective.
- Some experts think that eating fresh, oily fish more than once a week may protect against asthma.

Scientists have known for years that we all have millions of bacteria in our intestines. While some, like *E. coli*, can cause illness, others, like lactobacillus, are beneficial to health. But what do bugs in our gut have to do with asthma?

Swedish researchers compared gut microbes in allergic children from Sweden, a rich country with a high prevalence of allergy and nearby Estonia, a poor country with a low prevalence of allergy. Allergy was judged by a positive reaction to egg or cow's milk in a skin prick test. In both countries, allergic children had a higher rate of harmful gut bacteria and a lower rate of friendly gut bacteria.

Gut wars

At birth, a baby's gastrointestinal tract is sterile. Breastfeeding promotes the growth of good bacteria called lactobacilli. Potentially harmful bacteria are introduced from the environment. If the balance is right, the good bugs will balance out the bad bugs and keep the baby healthy. It seems that the first bacteria to arrive in the gut achieves a permanent territorial advantage. In Westernised societies, this can be hospital acquired organisms from procedures like Caesarean sections and special care units or a different microbial balance from baby formula rather than breastmilk.

Exclusive breastfeeding

A study of over 2,500 children in Western Australia from before birth to six years of age found that exclusive breastfeeding for at least four months provides protection against asthma at age six, as well as protection against lower respiratory tract illness and infections, ear infections and allergy. Exclusive breastfeeding means that the baby has never—not even once—taken any food other than breastmilk and that includes a bottle of cow's milk formula.

In Dunedin, New Zealand, a long-term study monitored 1,000 children for 25 years. Researchers found that children breastfed for four weeks or longer were more than twice as likely to develop asthma in mid-childhood, adolescence or young adulthood. However, the study didn't distinguish between breastfeeding and exclusive breastfeeding, because that wasn't an important issue 25 years ago.

> As it happens I had my first baby at Dunedin hospital. On the third day, when the baby had sucked all day and the milk hadn't arrived, the nurse "topped her up" with a bit of formula. I got the impression that this was a standard procedure.
> —*member of the failsafe email discussion groups*

Formula feeding

Although breast is best, some formulas promote a bowel microflora closer to that from breastmilk than others. Hydrolysed formulas have been found to produce a gut microflora more similar to that of breastfed babies than cow's milk formulas. In Canada, researchers checked on children who had been in an infant feeding study. They found that children who were exclusively breastfed or fed on a whey hydrolysate formula had a significantly lower incidence of asthma and eczema at age five than those fed on cow's milk or soy milk formula.

Raw farm milk

In Nepal, asthma researchers noticed that children were less likely to develop asthma when they were raised in houses where cattle were kept inside during the night. Numerous studies, mostly from Europe, reported similar protection from growing up on farms. But what is the protective factor?

A survey of farm children in Austria, Germany and Switzerland found that the only two protective factors were early exposure to stables and to raw farm milk. Before it is processed, milk contains a mixture of bacteria which will result in yoghurt if it is left to stand. The balance of bacteria is changed by pasteurisation. Researchers questioned more than 2,500 farming families. Children younger than a year old who were exposed to raw farm milk had lower frequencies of asthma. Continual long-term exposure to stables and farm milk until the age of five years was associated with the lowest frequencies of asthma. Protection seemed to begin while the mother was pregnant.

Pasteurisation was first introduced in the UK just over a hundred years ago. At first it was for the convenience of the producer, since pasteurisation (heating briefly to about 145°F) increased the shelf life of the milk. At that time, milk was often produced by diseased cattle in unsanitary conditions. Doctors soon realised that pasteurisation would rid milk of microbial contamination and bovine tuberculosis (TB). We now realise that pasteurisation also kills the good bacteria.

Antibiotics

Antibiotics are useful because they kill potentially harmful bacteria but the downside is that they also kill good bacteria as well. A number of studies have found that antibiotic treatment at birth inhibits the growth of good bacteria in babies' guts and encourages the growth of certain harmful bacteria by eliminating the competition.

A Belgian study examined antibiotic use in the first year of life. Rates of asthma and allergic disorders were compared in nearly 2,000 children, with and without antibiotics. The results were very clear. Hayfever in a parent is a strong risk factor for the development of asthma. For children *with* parental hayfever the *use of antibiotics in the first year of life was significantly related with later development of asthma* and eczema. There was no association in children *without* parental hayfever. In England, researchers looked at 25,000 children to investigate the effects of the mother's antibiotic use during pregnancy. Results suggested that the effects were related to dose—the more antibiotics the mother took, the higher the child's risk of developing asthma.

Experts now recommend minimising the use of antibiotics. For instance, most young children with ear infections will recover without the use of antibiotics. Treat only for pain, they say.

Probiotics

Traditionally, yoghurt was made by leaving fresh milk to stand for two days. The natural mixture of bacteria in the milk would create yoghurt. These good bugs are called probiotics. Modern food processing creates yoghurt by altering the bacterial balance of milk through pasteurisation then adding back a few probiotics in a sterile environment. These are not necessarily as effective as the originals.

Lactobacillus GG

A recently discovered probiotic called Lactobacillus GG appears to be particularly effective at colonising the human gut with friendly bacteria. It may even help to prevent asthma, according to a Finnish study published in the *Lancet*. Mothers at risk of having a baby with asthma were divided into groups. One group was given Lactobacillus GG in the last two weeks of their pregnancy and then for six months to the breastfeeding mothers or newborn babies. Eczema is the first allergic sign to emerge in the early years. After two years, 46 of the children had allergic eczema, six had asthma and one had hayfever. *The frequency of eczema in the probiotic group was half that of the control group.* Researchers stressed the necessity of very early intervention to make permanent changes in gut microflora. In older children and adults, continual supplementation will be needed.

Lactobacillus GG may reduce the need for antibiotics

In a study of more than 500 children in 18 Finnish day care centres, children were given milk with or without Lactobacillus GG for a period of seven months. Children in the Lactobacillus group had fewer days of absence from day care due to illness. There was also a reduction in the number of children suffering from respiratory infections with complications, lower respiratory tract infections, and the number of antibiotic treatments for respiratory tract infections. As a bonus, Lactobacillus GG was found to reduce the risk of dental caries.

Reducing diarrhoea

If you have to take antibiotics, then your gut microflora will be less disrupted if you can avoid antibiotic associated diarrhoea. Lactobacillus GG has been found to reduce the risk of antibiotic-associated diarrhoea in children so significantly it is now used as a treatment in some Australian hospitals.

Overall, Lactobacillus GG has been found to:
- colonise the gastrointestinal tract successfully
- reduce allergic conditions including asthma
- reduce colds, illnesses and dental caries in child care centres
- improve antibiotic-associated diarrhoea, travellers' diarrhoea and colitis
- reduce the severity and duration of infantile diarrhoea
- reduce inflammation and 'leaky gut' caused by rotavirus and cow's milk in patients sensitive to cow's milk
- reduce the number of tumours in rats with chemically induced colon cancer.

Testing so far has shown no adverse side effects.

Probiotics are big business

Lactobacillus GG was discovered in 1985 by Professor Sherwood Gorbach and Dr S Goldin from Tufts University School in Boston. Most of the research about Lactobacillus GG has originated either from these researchers or from researchers in Finland. You can see from author lists that these two groups work together. One of the papers from essentially the same set of researchers lists Valio Research and Development as their affiliation. In Australia, Lactobacillus GG is only available in Vaalia yoghurt produced by Pauls, a division of multinational food giant Parmalat. Pauls are the only company with the rights to use Lactobacillus GG in Australia.

It is ironic that simple bacteria which are freely available to the poorest peasant in the poorest countries in the world have ended up as profit-makers for some multinationals in Westernised societies. Nevertheless, I am convinced that Lactobacillus GG is worth a try, partly because of my own family's experience.

Probiotics and irritable bowel

After suffering for three years from gluten intolerance follow-ing a severe gastrointestinal infection, I experienced a remark-able improvement while trekking in Nepal. The Himalayan region has long been famous for the health giving properties of its fermented milk products and during a month's trek, I ate home-made yoghurt whenever possible. When we asked how the yoghurt was made, the instructions were simple: first, milk your buffalo, boil the milk, add starter, then let the milk stand for two days—in what we observed to be extremely unsterile conditions. It must have been crawling with bacteria, and it worked. Soon after the trek I passed a gluten challenge. Not long afterwards, our son suffered a bad bout of travellers' diarrhoea which resulted in gluten intolerance. By this time I had heard of Lactobacillus GG. After nearly a month of daily yoghurt, he too was able to eat wheat again. We are careful, switching to gluten free at the first sign of problems, and we eat Vaalia yoghurt as often as our dairy intolerance allows. For those who must avoid all dairy foods, Lactobacillus GG is avail-able in dairy-free capsules from the US, see p. 301.

The asthma–fish connection

There may be other foods which contribute to asthma preven-tion. Australian research in 1996 suggested that children who did not eat fish were three times more likely to develop asthma than children who ate fresh, oily fish more than once a week.

Although a similar study in Japan found the opposite—the risk of asthma increased with fish intake—Australian researchers think they are on to something. Studies which have focused on the use of fish oil supplements have not found significant improvement, except for a study of Japanese school-children which limited exposure to allergens as well as provid-ing fish oil supplements. A much larger study is currently underway in Australia, investigating the effects of dust mite control as well as dietary supplementation with capsules of tuna fish oil, in addition to cooking oils and margarines made from canola.

While we wait for results, and since fish is a healthy food, you might like to include at least two serves of fresh, oily fish in your weekly diet. By fresh, the researchers meant fish purchased fresh and uncooked. Oily fish were defined as more than 2 per cent fat and included silver bream, gemfish, mullet, orange roughy and rainbow trout. Canned fish did not have the same effect.

Conclusions

The lessons from this chapter seem clear. Lactobacillus GG has produced such positive results that its use has been accepted relatively quickly by the medical profession. We do not know yet whether probiotics can help adult asthmatics. It could be that very early doses give permanent protection for babies, while adults would need to eat yoghurt containing lactobacillus GG nearly every day. There are no apparent side effects. Fresh oily fish is a healthy food and, unless you are allergic to fish, there are no side effects.

If you come from a high risk family:
- breastfeed your baby
- include yoghurt containing Lactobacillus GG in your regular diet
- take Lactobacillus GG daily during late pregnancy and while breastfeeding
- avoid antibiotics unless absolutely necessary
- if you have to take antibiotics, take Lactobacillus GG as well
- include at least two serves of fresh fish in your weekly diet.

These measures do not guarantee asthma prevention, but they may give you a better chance.

13 Asthma in adults

Summary
- Asthma in adults can be a continuation of childhood asthma, a relapse of childhood asthma, or asthma experienced for the first time as an adult.
- Food and other chemicals can be associated with the development of asthma at any time.
- Women are more sensitive to food chemicals after the birth of their first child, pre-menstrually and when taking hormone replacement therapy.
- Occupational asthma is an important factor in adult-onset asthma. It is caused by hypersensitivity to an agent in the workplace.
- Workplace asthma can be difficult to identify. Symptoms can develop slowly. They will usually improve on weekends and holidays.
- Workplace asthma symptoms become irreversible with increasing exposure. The most effective treatment is to change jobs.
- Chemicals associated with workplace asthma can also affect people in the home environment.

Asthma is unpredictable. It can build up slowly or start as a severe attack at any age. One man who had grown out of childhood asthma at the age of 16 developed asthma again as an adult. His first attack after 20 asthma-free years was sudden and frightening. 'I didn't know what was happening. I think some people must die of fear,' he said.

An estimated 10 per cent of adults in Australia are asthmatics. About 80 per cent of adults with persistant asthma have reduced lung function. One in four avoid socialising in smoky restaurants, pubs and clubs.

Could it be food?

Remember the woman on p. 38 who switched to diet cola because she wanted to lose weight? One little change in her diet was enough to initiate adult-onset asthma induced by the preservative sodium benzoate. Although she never saw an obvious reaction, all she had to do was switch back to regular cola and her asthma went away again.

WHO IS MOST SENSITIVE TO FOOD CHEMICALS?
- children
- women of childbearing age
- the elderly

Men in the prime of their lives are least likely to be affected

WHAT FACTORS CAN INCREASE YOUR CHANCE OF BEING AFFECTED?
- exposure to toxic chemicals
- increased intake of additives or other food chemicals
- illnesses like giardia and rotavirus
- hormones

Hormones can make you more sensitive

Women who are sensitive to foods are at their most sensitive when premenstrual. This is the time when they need to be most careful about avoiding food chemicals to which they react.

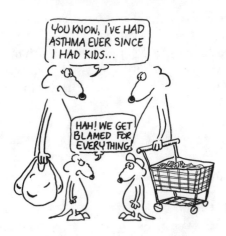

There are a number of accounts of severe asthma attacks linked with menstruation.

Women also face hormonal changes during pregnancy and breastfeeding. Many mothers later realise that their food intolerance symptoms dated from the birth of their first child. When they go on the diet, their symptoms—including asthma— improve for the first time in years. Remember the nurse on p. 70? Her asthma started as cough following respiratory tract infections 'while I was having my babies'. It wasn't until she did the diet for her children's behaviour that the causes of her asthma became obvious.

Hormone replacement therapy (HRT)

Among the long-term adverse effects of HRT is a possible connection between HRT and asthma. A 10-year study by researchers at Harvard Medical School found that high doses of hormone therapy increased the risk of asthma in post-menopausal users, and long-term use of 10-years or more at any time of life doubled the risk of asthma.

Occupational asthma

Work can be an important cause of adult-onset asthma. Occupational asthma is caused by hypersensitivity to a sensitising agent in the workplace. Symptoms can develop quickly or slowly. It can be difficult to recognise the symptoms as occupational asthma while the condition is still reversible.

A woman describes her father's occupational asthma:

> Dad worked for a chemical company all his working life. They knew the chemicals caused his asthma, but they wouldn't admit it. After years of fighting, they gave him compensation but it was too late. He had no quality of life for the last 10 years. He couldn't breathe.

There is always a period, from weeks to years, at the beginning of the job when the worker is free of symptoms. Recurrent hayfever during working hours can be the first sign of problems. This is followed by increasing cough perhaps with chest tightness. Wheeze and breathlessness usually come later.

The most obvious feature of occupational asthma is the timing. If symptoms occur within a short time after exposure, diagnosis is easy. More commonly, symptoms develop four to eight hours after the start of the shift and increase after the end of the shift. The worker might experience his worst symptoms at home, or wake with a night cough. At first, symptoms will occur only during the working week, worsening towards the end of the week and improving during weekends and holidays.

If exposure continues, symptoms will stop improving during breaks from work. Extra symptoms will develop, most

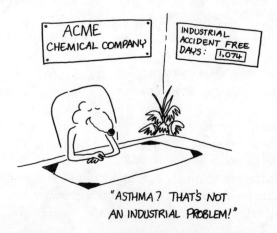

"ASTHMA? THAT'S NOT AN INDUSTRIAL PROBLEM!"

commonly breathlessness on exertion. The asthma will stop being occupational and become permanent.

Medication is only a short-term treatment for occupational asthma. *The most effective treatment is for the worker to avoid exposure by changing jobs.* If this happens while symptoms are still improving on weekends, the asthma will usually disappear over a period of weeks or months. If the worker stays on the job despite symptoms there is a very real risk that asthma will last for years, or permanently, when he or she finally leaves the job. By this time the asthma will be the same as non-occupational asthma and may be sensitive to other triggers.

SOME CAUSES OF OCCUPATIONAL ASTHMA

Occupational asthma has been associated with:

- chemicals such as isocyanates (used by spray painters, polyurethane foam manufacturers), aluminium smelting fumes, curing agents for epoxy resins and paints, fumes from soldering and welding, phthalic anhydride used in the chemical industry and by plastics manufacturers and many others
- pesticides used by farmers
- animal and insect proteins—from horses to laboratory rats to mites in cereal grains
- flour dust and other foods
- hundreds of other agents, including antibiotics and medications in pharmaceutical manufacturing, dyes used by textile and food workers, latex used by health care workers and enzymes in washing powders.

Anyone can be affected

You don't have to be a worker to develop asthma from exposure to these substances.

In Madrid, Spain, a two-year-old boy developed asthma, urticaria and dermatitis over a period of 12 months when visiting his grandfather's bakery. At the end of that time he would develop asthma after playing with flour for 10 minutes. Doctors concluded he had 'the childhood equivalent of occupational bakers' asthma'.

Two patients from the thoracic unit at St Vincents Hospital in Sydney illustrate the effects of organophosphate insectides. A 21-year-old man with a 10-year history of mild asthma developed increasing afternoon breathlessness over six months. At the abattoir where he worked he had been moved to a job supervising storage of sheep skins. He showed no reaction to sheep, but the skins were sprayed once a month with an organophosphate insecticide. Tests revealed a delayed reaction starting after two hours and peaking six hours later. When moved to a different section of the abattoir, his symptoms improved.

The second patient was a 52-year-old woman who had developed asthma for the first time in her life six months previously. Her symptoms sometimes seemed worse when her cat was around. Just as well she didn't give her cat away—an alert doctor realised that she had no reaction to cat dander and arranged for a flea collar to be left in the room with her without her knowledge. She was found to react to an insecticide in the collar, and was advised to remove the cat collar and pest strips in her home. Over the next three months, her symptoms improved.

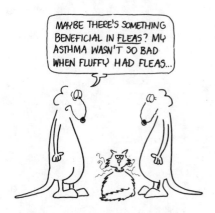

How many have occupational asthma?
It is generally estimated that about 10 per cent of asthma in adults is caused by their work. In Finland, it is easier to calculate

a more precise figure because asthmatics have to register for medication rebates. A 12-year study published in 2001 surveyed Finnish adults aged 25–59. Work-related asthma was found *in nearly 30 per cent of the asthmatic men and 20 per cent of the asthmatic women.* The researchers concluded that the impact of occupational exposure in the start of adult-onset persistent asthma is 'much larger and more widely spread than generally assumed'.

If you have developed adult onset asthma, consider your job—does the timing suggest occupational asthma?—and consider what you eat. Major changes of diet can happen with a move, a student leaving home, a new partner, a holiday, increasing affluence or a weight loss diet. Sometimes one tiny change is all it takes—such as switching to a diet drink, or consuming more wine. Don't think you will see an obvious reaction. If you notice any effect at all, it is usually the tip of the iceberg.

14 Asthma and Australian Aborigines

Summary

- Some experts say that Aborigines have a natural immunity to asthma.
- Recent studies and Aboriginal health care workers do not agree.
- There is considerable variation between Aboriginal children living in the most remote outstations and living in towns. Aboriginal children in towns have the same prevalence of asthma as non-Aboriginal children.
- Aboriginal people themselves call asthma 'short wind'.
- The Short Wind project provides culturally sensitive asthma education resources that deal with the special problems faced by Aboriginal asthmatics.

Experts disagree about asthma among Aborigines. Some say that Aborigines have a natural immunity to asthma. Others say this is a myth. One study found Aboriginal children living in rural towns had the same prevalence of asthma as non-Aboriginal children. Another found Aboriginal children in remote communities had the same prevalence, although an earlier study found much lower rates of asthma, particularly in 'outstations' in Central Australia where small groups of several families live in remote desert locations on or near traditional lands.

Aboriginal health

Studies in Western Australia's remote desert areas show that, despite improvements, Aboriginal babies have higher rates of infant mortality, failure to thrive and undernutrition than other parts of Australia. Aboriginal children have higher rates of respiratory, gastrointestinal and other infections. Aboriginal adults are prone to obesity, high blood pressure, adult-onset diabetes and cardiovascular diseases.

The poor health of Aboriginal people is related to underemployment, overcrowding, limited education, inadequate housing, a high rate of smoking, alcohol abuse, petrol sniffing, inadequate nutrition and a low rate of breastfeeding. Some communities are situated in dusty, fly-ridden locations with little access to washing facilities. Access to health care is poor. Virtually all children in remote communities have a profuse, chronic nasal discharge.

In the clinics

Meanwhile, people who work with Aborigines see asthma as a major health problem. There is a high demand for asthma medications. With Aboriginal people forming 25 per cent of her case load, Darwin asthma educator Jan Saunders was frustrated by the inadequacy of current asthma management resources:

How could I explain asthma management to someone who spoke English as a second or even a third language? Our current brochures were written for people with a high degree of literacy and weren't very colourful or pictorial. Use of an interpreter was not an option . . . there are at least 100 different dialects across the Top End of the Northern Territory alone.

The Short Wind project

Jan's frustration led to a project providing culturally sensitive education resources about basic asthma-prevention hygiene and the use of asthma medications. 'I quickly discovered that symptoms such as "shortness of breath" meant nothing to Aboriginal people,' said Jan. 'Aboriginal health workers suggested I ask Aboriginal clients if they have "short wind" instead. This proved so successful that "Short Wind" was kept as the title for the project.'

Carried out by Asthma NT, the Danila Dilba Aboriginal medical services and Flinders University School of Nursing, the Short Wind project provides culturally sensitive flipcharts, posters, T-shirts, asthma plans and calico carry bags to meet the needs of Aboriginal people.

Materials in the Short Wind project deal with difficulties facing asthmatics in Aboriginal communities. The message is basically take your asthma medication, eat healthy food, get plenty of exercise and don't smoke.

There are also tips about health and hygiene regarding asthma prevention which provide a glimpse of the problems facing Aboriginal families.

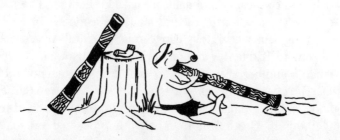

- **Colds and flu**
  Wash hands often.
  Wash cups and dishes often.
  Eat healthy foods including bush tucker.
  Cover mouth when coughing.
- **Camp fire smoke especially wood from mangrove trees**
  Try not to have camp fires near the house or near children.
- **Exercise**
  When hunting, gathering food or exercising always carry blue reliever puffer.
- **Pollens, moulds, animal hair**
  Try not to sleep next to the dogs and cats.
  Try to keep dogs and cats out of the house.
  Try to wash clothing weekly.
  Keep the house clean.
  Keep away from strong smelling trees and bushes.
- **Dust and dust mites**
  Take away old mattresses, pillows and old clothing.
  Hang sheets and blankets in the sun to kill dust mites.
  Water down dust near the house.

(Edited extract from the Short Wind project, with permission)

Bush tucker and community stores

The traditional diet of bush tucker is of course additive-free and extremely healthy but this is only a proportion of what Aborigines eat. The rest is highly processed food. The proportion of bush tucker to processed food varies widely between communities. Aborigines most likely to eat a high proportion of bush tucker are those in outstations which are chosen for their location on or near traditional lands used for hunting. This could account for variations in the prevalence of asthma.

During four-wheel drive trips through Central Australia and the remote Kimberley region of Western Australia, we have visited a number of the more accessible Aboriginal communities. The community stores always shock me. There is usually almost nothing in them that I am prepared to eat myself or feed my children. Most of the food is highly processed and loaded with additives. In one store, one-eighth of the entire food display consisted of two litre containers of highly coloured, sulphite and benzoate-preserved fruit flavoured cordials.

It is an open secret that foods destined for the far north of Australia—especially the cheaper brands—often contain higher than legal limits of preservatives because manufacturers want products to last in the harsh climate and know that they are extremely unlikely to be caught.

Over the years that I have given talks in the Northern Territory, I have been approached many times by health workers who are horrified by the foods in Aboriginal communities. They are the very worst processed foods: cheap, high fat, high salt, high sugar, high additive and lacking in nutrition.

Diet makes a difference

I have worked with a few urban Aboriginal children with behaviour problems. One boy had been referred to a doctor with suspected ADHD. Most of his diet was failsafe. Dinner was usually meat stew and rice. After school he had additive-laden snacks and drinks. I asked his mother what she ate at his age. Damper with golden syrup. Right, I suggested, give him that. His behaviour changed overnight.

The causes of ill health and asthma in Aborigines are a complicated combination in which food additives are a tiny factor. It is unrealistic to expect Aboriginal families either to go back to their traditional bush tucker diet or to avoid additives. They just don't have access to suitable food. Removing sulphites and colours from processed foods would be one small positive step.

15 Worst case scenario: anaphylaxis

Summary
- Anaphylaxis is the most severe of the allergic disorders, resulting in a sudden, potentially fatal, widespread reaction that can involve breathing, itching, rash, swelling, diarrhoea, shock and heart attack.
- The prevalence of anaphylaxis is increasing dramatically.
- Asthmatics with a history of allergy have the highest risk of anaphylactic reactions.
- The main triggers for anaphylaxis are medications, food and insect stings. Anaphylaxis triggers can be associated with less severe asthmatic reactions.
- Latex allergy is a new and increasing source of anaphylaxis.
- The best way to prevent anaphylaxis is allergen avoidance.
- Asthmatics need to know how to recognise an anaphylactic reaction and what to do about it.

Anaphylaxis is a worst-case scenario for asthmatics. The most severe of the allergic disorders, it is a sudden, potentially fatal, widespread reaction that can involve various systems of the body including the respiratory tract, skin, gastrointestinal tract, and cardiovascular system. Reactions in at least two systems—such as asthma plus hives—are usually required for a diagnosis of anaphylaxis.

Symptoms usually occur within minutes to two hours after contact with the trigger although occasionally reactions may occur up to six hours later. Reactions can be *bi-phasic*, that is, the first reaction is followed by recovery then a second reaction some hours later, possibly worse than the first.

Anaphylactic reactions can be mild to life-threatening. The most serious is *anaphylactic shock*, a widespread reaction which causes swelling, constriction of the airways, heart failure, circulatory collapse, and sometimes death.

Although it is called an allergic disorder, an anaphylactic reaction is not always a true allergy. Reactions to medications, additives and salicylates are often intolerance reactions rather than immune (IgE) responses.

Asthmatics with a history of allergy have a particularly high risk of developing anaphylactic reactions, especially women of child-bearing age.

Anaphylaxis is increasing

Until recently anaphylaxis was regarded as rare, but the prevalence of anaphylaxis is increasing in Westernised countries. In Brisbane, Australia, a survey conducted over a full year in an adult emergency department in the late 1990s found approximately 0.2 per cent of patients admitted with anaphylaxis. This was higher than expected. One patient died following a bee sting. About 30 per cent were related to drugs, and 20 per cent each to food and insects. For the rest, causes were unknown. Half of all cases were classified as severe anaphylaxis. A quarter of the patients were asthmatics.

Foods

Death from food reactions is usually caused by breathing difficulties that can lead to respiratory arrest within 30 minutes. People with a family history of allergy, bronchial asthma and prior allergic reactions to food are at a particularly high risk.

Foods most often associated with anaphylaxis are peanuts and tree nuts especially in children and young adults, and fish and crustaceans (shrimp, prawn, scallop and crab but not lobster).

The Brisbane adult study listed fish and seafood (13 cases), nuts (4), fruit drinks (2) and other foods (3). Many foods— including egg, milk and soy—and additives such as colours and sulphites can be associated with anaphylaxis.

Food-dependent exercise-induced anaphylaxis is rare but increasing. The reaction is caused by the combination of food plus exercise, which can be as little as a brisk walk a few hours after eating. The condition can be hard to diagnose because neither the food alone nor the exercise alone will provoke the symptoms. People with this kind of reaction typically have asthma. It is usually not a true allergy and avoidance of aspirin and other non-steroidal anti-inflammatory drugs (NSAIDs) is often recommended. Foods such as wheat, gluten, fish, milk and fruit have been associated with this condition, but it seems likely that the contribution of salicylates in foods has been underestimated (see p. 144).

Avoidance

The best way to prevent anaphylaxis is to avoid your triggering food, but this can be very difficult. Medical journals contain numerous reports of severe anaphylactic reactions to tiny quantities of allergens hidden in processed food or encountered in unexpected ways.

FROM THE MEDICAL JOURNALS
- In the US, two young children reacted to 'dairy–free' sorbets contaminated by milk products when manufactured in machinery used also to make icecream.

- In Australia, two egg–sensitive children reacted with anaphylaxis when a powdered egg white pavlova mix was opened and transferred to a bowl in the same room as the child.
- In Europe, doctors complained about anaphylaxis resulting from the hidden peanut content of American and Asian cuisines, including peanut oil in pizza sauce.

Anaphylactic reaction in a medical student

An asthmatic medical student (MS) was rushed to hospital when he experienced hives, severe tightening of his throat and shortness of breath while eating dinner. His next attack happened five weeks later while MS was on rounds at the hospital. He was immediately admitted as a patient. His breakfast had been a glass of orange juice and three yellow jelly beans. His condition fluctuated and eventually staff realised worsening symptoms were associated with a drug. When the drug was withdrawn, MS recovered. The drug was coloured with tartrazine 102 (yellow #5), and was also in the jelly beans. Dinner had been a bright orange-yellow cauliflower cheese. Since then, 'in spite of careful screening by an alert, educated patient', MS has suffered two more moderate attacks after eating foods later found to contain tartrazine.

Anaphylaxis from mould in a pancake mix

Penicillin is the single most common cause of anaphylaxis. A college student (CS) with a history of asthma and allergies to pets, moulds, and penicillin had pancakes for breakfast. The packaged mix had been opened and stored for about two years. CS ate two pancakes which tasted like 'rubbing alcohol'. Minutes later he became short of breath. Rushed to a nearby clinic, he was able to walk in but suddenly collapsed in cardiopulmonary arrest. The pancake mix contained a high mould count including penicillin. It seems that CS died from a reaction to penicillin mould.

Drugs

Anaphylactic reactions to drugs and latex have increased because the use of drugs and latex have increased. The drugs listed below are the most likely to cause anaphylaxis.

ANTIBIOTICS

Antibiotics including penicillin and cephalosporins are considered to have the biggest potential to cause anaphylaxis. A life-long asthmatic took her prescription to a pharmacy. Instead of an antibiotic which she had taken safely many times before, the pharmacist offered a generic alternative, 'exactly the same but cheaper'. When she took the first capsule, she was alone at home. Within minutes she developed itching, hives and breathing difficulty. Being close to the hospital, she dashed to her car and set out. By the time she arrived, her face was so swollen she could hardly see, she was gasping for breath and bright red all over. Driving up to the front door of the hospital, she leaned on the horn and collapsed while staff came running.

NSAIDS

Aspirin and the other NSAIDs have long been known to cause adverse effects. A centre in Holland which monitors reports of adverse reactions to drugs warns that there is a relatively high risk of developing an anaphylactic reaction during the use of NSAIDs, especially ibuprofen, naproxen and diclofenac. When a new and quite different NSAID called celecoxib was released, researchers hoped it would have fewer side-effects. Within a short time, a doctor's wife experienced acute itching, hives,

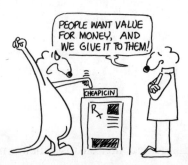

respiratory distress, a drop in blood pressure and collapse within 15 minutes of taking one capsule. She had taken the drug six months previously for tendonitis without difficulty. The woman had no previous history of allergy, asthma or adverse reactions to drugs. Asthmatics should approach NSAIDs with caution. See p. 86 for more information.

ANAESTHETICS

Anaphylaxis during operations is commonly reported. While anaesthetics are usually blamed for this, a Sydney review of 23 heart-surgery patients who experienced anaphylactic reactions during surgery found that the majority reacted to antibiotics (30 per cent) and gelatin solutions (25 per cent). Drugs are administered not only by mouth or injection. Anaphylaxis has been reported in a number of children due to gelatin coating on rectal suppositories used to administer drugs.

RADIOCONTRAST DYES

Isosulfan blue is one of a number of dyes used because they will show up on X-rays. It is used during mapping of lymph nodes in the management of high-risk melanoma and other cancers. Of 250 patients exposed to this dye, 2 per cent developed anaphylaxis and a further 3 per cent developed blue hives.

SULPHITE PRESERVATIVES IN DRUGS

A drug monitoring system in Colorado lists reports of anaphylactic or asthmatic reactions associated with sulphite-containing local anaesthetics, gentamicin, metoclopramide, doxycycline and vitamin B complex. Reactions to sulphites in injectible drugs are quicker than those caused by sulphites in foods. Patients with a history of sulphite reactions may be at increased risk but those without such a history may also react. Sulphite-free alternatives should be used if available.

IMMUNOTHERAPY

With immunotherapy, patients are given small but increasing doses of an allergen to densensitise their immune systems and stop asthma attacks. Occasionally, patients suffer life-threatening anaphylactic shock from this therapy.

Latex

Allergy to natural rubber latex is a newly recognised health hazard presented to the medical profession by the US Food and Drug Administration (FDA) in 1992. Latex allergy can lead to chronic occupational asthma, anaphylaxis, and even death. Since 1989, the FDA has received reports of more than 1,100 injuries and 15 deaths. People with frequent exposure to latex—such as health care workers and hospital patients—are the most likely to develop sensitivity. Reactions to latex can be true allergies or a delayed hypersensitivity reaction. The latter is more common, the former is more life-threatening. Powder-free gloves or washing the powder from gloves can reduce the risk because latex proteins bind to the glove powder and are then easily inhaled.

Sensitisation can occur during surgery, dental work and internal examinations when the latex protein comes in contact with mucous membranes. A woman who entered hospital with suspected premature labour experienced an anaphylactic reaction to latex minutes after an internal examination. With the baby in fetal distress, she was rushed into an emergency Caesarian operation.

In Italy, a 5–year–old girl suffered anaphylaxis after playing in a ball pit at a fast–food outlet. Two months later, a 9–year–old boy had an asthma attack with loss of consciousness while playing in the playpen of a different outlet belonging to the same company. Although the balls were not made of latex, they were found to be contaminated with latex from the lining of the ball pit.

Latex and food

Certain fruits including bananas, kiwi fruit and avocados have cross reactivity with latex. After ten years working in hospitals, a German nurse developed conjunctivitis, rhinitis and shortness of breath while wearing latex gloves. One night, minutes after snacking on banana and kiwi fruit, he was called to a patient. Starting with itchy feet and hands, his symptoms progressed rapidly to a medical emergency involving severe breathlessness. The fruit was considered to be a possible booster to the latex in his gloves and the air in the emergency room.

Early recognition of latex allergy is important. An Australian critical care nurse suffered increasingly severe asthma, urticaria (hives) and oedema (fluid retention) for five years before being diagnosed with latex allergy. By that time, she had become so sensitive that even inhaled fumes could trigger an anaphylactic reaction.

Insect bites

Anaphylactic reactions to venom are most likely to involve shock and in fatal cases the average time to cardiac arrest is 15 minutes. Although bee, wasp and hornet stings are the most commonly involved, some regions have their own specialty. In Brisbane, a tick commonly associated with paralysis in animals has been linked with anaphylaxis in humans and a caterpillar has also been reported.

Although in other categories of anaphylaxis, the patient is most likely to be a female of child-bearing age with a history of allergy, people who actually die from insect stings are most likely to be non-allergic males.

To minimise the risk of an insect sting, when outside avoid brightly coloured clothing or scented toiletries which will attract insects. Avoid walking barefoot on lawns where there may be bees and keep insecticide close when cooking or working outdoors. In Darwin, a tragic accident shocked the community when a fit, young council worker encountered a wasp nest in a tree while carrying out repairs. He died within minutes from receiving hundreds of stings while his co-workers ran for insecticide.

Unknown causes

Anaphylaxis of unknown origin (called *idiopathic*) is a dangerous situation, because reactions can happen again at any time. About a third of all anaphylactic reactions are in this category. It seems likely that at least some of these cases might be related to hidden food chemicals including salicylates in foods, see p. 144.

Management of frequent episodes is with daily preventive medication, corticosteroids, antihistamines and bronchodilators. Management of infrequent episodes is treatment of attacks when they occur. One study showed that people with idiopathic anaphylaxis were much better at carrying a self-injecting adrenaline pen at all times than those who knew the cause of their anaphylaxis.

Use of an elimination diet to reveal a food trigger

Allergy testing is traditionally used to identify food triggers of anaphylaxis but with salicylates or a food additive where the response is not a true allergy, allergy testing is useless. An elimination diet can be used. If challenges are to be carried out they must be carefully administered by experts within a hospital environment.

A 22-year-old healthy male (HM) experienced anaphylactic reactions several times a year for four years. Within 10 minutes of eating certain foods he would develop flushing, difficulty breathing, nausea, vomiting, swelling of the face and tongue, and loss of consciousness. Suspect foods included pizza, barbecue chicken, cola, garlic bread, beer, gravy and Chinese takeaway. After following a strict elimination diet for four weeks, HM took challenge capsules which showed a mild asthmatic reaction with tongue swelling to both colours and sulphites and an urticarial rash to salicylates. A severe anaphylactic reaction occurred 15 minutes after both sodium nitrate and sodium nitrite challenges. These preservatives are used in processed meats such as bacon, ham, salami and corned beef. After three and a half years on a diet free of nitrates, nitrites, sulphites and low in salicylates, HM has had no further reactions.

Anaphylaxis caused by salicylates in foods

While the anaphylaxis-causing potential for salicylates in aspirin and NSAIDs is one of the best documented in all of the medical literature, there is almost nothing about salicylates in foods. It may seem impossible that people could develop anaphylaxis from a chemical in a wide range of common foods we all eat every day. Yet some people have just that—salicylate-induced anaphylaxis.

> My friend has life-threatening anaphylactic reactions to salicylates in drugs and food. Since following the failsafe diet she has had only one small reaction (and she admits to 'cheating' that day) in the last 11 months. Before that, she was speeding to the hospital in an ambulance about every 10–14 days. She has also reduced the antihistamines that she takes by more than half . . . Her own allergy doctor is very impressed with her current health. It seems weird that she has had to find her own help and that doctors seem to have little knowledge of her allergy to natural aspirin. Now I don't fear for her safety because the life threatening reactions have disappeared.
> —*from the US*

Management

The best way to manage anaphylaxis is avoidance of triggers. Hospital treatment consists of adrenaline, antihistamines and corticosteroids as required. Some experts recommend that anyone who has had an attack of life-threatening anaphylaxis should carry a self-injecting adrenaline pen. Choose one without sulphite preservatives. A study of US fatalities showed that adolescents who have peanut and tree nut allergy and asthma and don't have quick access to these devices are at highest risk for a fatal reaction because they are more likely to eat away from home, they are less likely to carry medications, and may ignore or not recognise symptoms.

An Australian teenager was just 17 when he started on his first day of work experience. Not wanting to be different, he bought his lunch at the same take-away counter as his new work mates. He had a known allergy to peanuts but presumably he thought a burger was safe so he didn't ask. There was peanut in the sauce and he died within minutes.

HOW DOES IT FEEL?
An anaphylactic reaction may begin with:
- a tingling sensation, itching, metallic taste in the mouth
Other symptoms can include:
- hives, a sensation of warmth, asthma symptoms, swelling of the mouth and throat area, difficulty breathing, vomiting, diarrhoea, cramping, a drop in blood pressure, and loss of consciousness.

Symptoms may begin in as little as 5 to 15 minutes to up to two hours after exposure to the allergen, but life–threatening reactions may progress over hours.

An English survey of 70 anaphylactic reactions which should have benefited from self-injecting pens found only half had used their adrenaline. Of those, 20 per cent claimed immediate benefit and 10 per cent claimed no benefit. The other half did not have their kit at the time or preferred to get medical assistance. The researcher concluded that, rather than rescue by adrenaline kit, management might be better directed towards effective allergen avoidance.

WHAT TO DO IF YOU HAVE AN ANAPHYLACTIC REACTION
Act quickly
- Recognise symptoms.
- Get to hospital as quickly as possible (do not drive yourself) or phone an ambulance and ask for adrenaline.
- Stay in hospital at least six hours because sometimes there is a second reaction. Sit in the lobby reading a magazine if necessary.

Ask for a referral to an allergist to confirm your trigger
- If the trigger is not revealed by allergy testing, consider the failsafe diet supervised by an experienced dietitian with careful challenges in hospital.

Carry a sulphite–free self–injecting adrenaline pen at all times
- Teach yourself and others how to use it by practising often with an expired pen on an orange.
- Wear a medical bracelet.

16 Breathing lessons

Summary
- Some asthmatics may have disordered breathing patterns.
- There is a small but growing body of scientific evidence that a range of breathing therapies, including the Buteyko breathing technique, can lead to a reduction of medication use in asthma.
- Buteyko practitioners also recommend avoidance of certain foods.
- Since funding for asthma research often comes from drug companies, researchers have difficulty obtaining funding for non-drug treatments for asthma.

A few years ago, Michael Cichorski was marketing manager for asthma medications at a pharmaceutical company with annual sales of more than $50 billion. As an asthmatic since the age of seven, Cichorski was not only selling asthma drugs, he was also using them.

'I was taking more and more medications—both the puffers for relief and the steroids used for prevention, but if I stopped them, the asthma came back,' he told *Australian Financial Review* journalist Ray Moynihan. 'I was concerned I was building a life-long dependency on very potent medications.' As an employee of a large drug company, Cichorski had easy access to the medical literature about drugs. He wasn't concerned about the effectiveness of the drugs but, reading the literature, he became more and more worried about potential side effects, particularly with long-term usage.

Then Cichorski accepted a challenge from a Buteyko practitioner. Despite being sceptical, after just five sessions he was able to dramatically reduce his reliever medications. Within six months, he had stopped using steroids as well. Now he describes himself as 'drug free and asthma free'. He has left the drug industry for a new career as a Buteyko practitioner.

The Buteyko breathing technique was developed in 1952 by a Russian doctor who noticed that healthy subjects breathing deeply for some time would become dizzy, wheeze, cough and eventually faint. Dr Buteyko developed a system of shallow breathing to correct the problems in people with disordered breathing patterns, including asthmatics. Despite strong opposition from doctors at first, news of the effective therapy was spread by successful patients and clinics sprang up all over the world.

The hyperventilation syndrome

While Dr Buteyko was working in Russia, Western doctors had discovered a similar condition called hyperventilation syndrome, estimating that this syndrome contributes to 10 per cent of all out-patient referrals to hospital.

Additives to Avoid card

Pop out and keep handy in wallet

ADDITIVES TO AVOID

Artificial colours

102	tartrazine
104	quinoline yellow
110	sunset yellow
122	carmoisine
123	amaranth
124	ponceau
127	erythrosine
129	allura red

132	indigotine
133	brilliant blue
142	food green
143	fast green
151	brilliant black
155	chocolate brown

Natural colour

160b	annatto

Preservatives

200–203 sorbic acid and sorbates

210–213 benzoic acid and benzoates

220–228 sulphur dioxide and sulphites

280–283 propionic acid and propionates

249–252 nitrates, nitrites

Antioxidants

310–312 gallates

319 TBHQ

320 BHA

321 BHT

Flavour enhancers

620–625 Glutamates, MSG, HVP, HPP

627 Disodium guanylate

631 Disodium inosinate

635 Ribonucleotides

SOME SIGNS OF HYPERVENTILATION DISORDER
- Constricted chest, shortness of breath, accelerated or deepened breathing, unable to breathe deeply, chest pain, feeling tense, palpitations.
- Tightness around the mouth, stiffness of fingers or arms, cold hands or feet, tingling fingers.
- Dizzy spells, blurred vision, being confused.

Some 30–40 per cent of asthmatics may have disordered breathing, according to two British studies. Since the only way to confirm dysfunctional breathing is by successful treatment with breathing therapy, they recommended that facilities for breathing therapy should be available as part of the overall management of asthmatic patients.

A range of breathing therapies for hyperventilation and yoga breathing techniques, such as Sahaja meditation, have been found to make patients feel better, but two Australian studies suggest that the Buteyko method may be more effective at achieving a reduction in medication use.

The Mater study
In a study at the Brisbane Mater hospital, 19 asthma patients attending classes with a Buteyko instructor reduced their use of bronchodilators—but not steroids—by about 90 per cent. This was significantly better than the control group who took asthma education classes which included general relaxation techniques and conventional breathing exercises and achieved a 5 per cent drop in medication use.

The Monash video study
At Monash Medical School in Melbourne, a group of 18 asthmatics learned their breathing exercises from a video watched at home twice a day for four weeks. They were able to reduce their use of inhaled bronchodilator medications by an average of 60 per cent, compared to a control group who watched a nature video.

The full Buteyko video took 67 minutes. It contained explanations of theory as well as 20 minutes of a self-guided session. There was also a manual. On average, subjects watched the 20 minute video session 37 times.

Did they change their diet?
Advice was provided on the video about dietary changes, medication usage and how to control allergic responses. Subjects were neither encouraged or discouraged regarding changing their diets. Whether they did so was not recorded.

There was a marked and significant decrease in the use of inhaled bronchodilator medications and a significant improvement in quality of life—twice as great as that achieved by conventional asthma education in a Royal Prince Alfred Hospital (RPAH) outpatients clinic study, noted the researchers.

Despite significant reductions in medication and improvement in quality of life, patients showed no improvement on the standard lung function tests in either trial. I suggest that the Buteyko method would be most effective when combined with the failsafe diet.

Will breath training help you?
Try this simple Buteyko test. Sit down and breathe through your nose for two minutes. Breathe out completely, squeezing your nose to block it and start timing yourself. At the first sign of discomfort, start breathing again and write down the time achieved. This is called your control pause. A reading of 60 is perfect. A reading of 40–60 seconds is normal. A reading of less than 30 seconds and especially 15 seconds or less suggests you will benefit from classes.

The technique focuses on learning shallow breathing and on increasing the length of both the control pause described above, and the maximum pause, which is the longest time you can hold your breath out. The Butyeko method can be learned from a video or with expert supervision. When the technique is perfected, the maximum pause is regarded as equivalent to one puff of bronchodilator medication. It is used as part of a routine: one

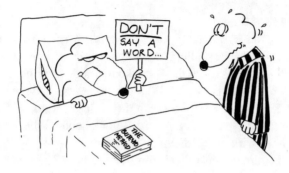

maximum pause, three minutes shallow breathing, one maximum pause. If this is not effective, bronchodilator medication is used.

One aspect of the Buteyko method which can deter parents is the practice of taping the mouth while sleeping to promote nose breathing. For a first person account of this experience, see the box below.

REPORT FROM A BUTEYKO GRADUATE

Taping the mouth closed while you sleep is not dangerous. I was told to use Micropore tape, through which you can actually breathe if you try hard enough, and which will come unstuck if you force your mouth open, however I have never had to do this.

After almost a year of taping my mouth, I find that I sleep with my mouth shut now without it. However if my nose is at all runny or blocked or I am even the slightest bit wheezy, I tape it to make sure that I don't go back to my old ways. While taping your mouth is a pretty weird thing to do (my husband certainly thought so until he saw the improvements), to me it is definitely preferable to all the side effects from the large doses of bronchodilators I used to need on a daily basis.

Buteyko students are also taught that some foods interfere with breathing. The list of prohibited foods appears to depend on the individual practitioner. The Buteyko graduate above was given a list of foods which meant avoiding additives, some high salicylate foods and some allergens.

The results

A letter in the *Medical Journal of Australia* written by staff at a Melbourne hospital allergy clinic described one woman's remarkable success with the Buteyko method. Their patient was a 40-year-old woman with life-long asthma who had previously required use of her puffer once a day unless she took a beclomethasone preventer daily. After a Buteyko course she managed her asthma without medication for more than five years, and reported 'tremendous relief' from the method. The patient had a known sensitivity to horse hair and on three occasions developed severe bronchoconstriction after exposure to horses. She carried her puffer as recommended and only one of these episodes resulted in urgent hospitalisation. The other two settled easily after she used her puffer.

More details

The Buteyko technique is not suitable for children under the age of four. It is expensive, costing hundreds of dollars for about five sessions, although this isn't a lot compared to a lifetime of doctors' consultations and medication. The video is cheaper and has a money-back guarantee. See p. 300 for details about contacting a Buteyko practitioner or buying the video.

Profits and funding

Asthma drugs are a massive $300 million annual market. Sales of puffers in Australia are worth $80 million a year.

If results like those achieved in the Melbourne and Brisbane Buteyko studies could be achieved in the general population, and breathing classes were more widely adopted, drug companies would experience a loss in profits. Does this affect the 'best practice' medicine offered to patients? Simple non-drug treatments for asthma such as diet and breathing lessons do not feature in routine asthma management.

In Australia, most of the funding for asthma research comes from the manufacturers of asthma medications. Those companies would have little interest in a technique which doesn't

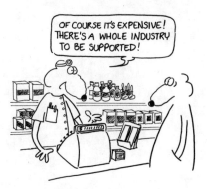

involve medications and which may result in fewer medications needed.

For example, the Monash Buteyko trial had difficulty attracting funds and was done without any external funding, relying almost entirely on the hard work of student and lead author, Ashley Opat. In Brisbane, the Mater study was funded by the Australian Association of Asthma Foundations.

I would be pleased to see breathing classes cheaply and easily available to every asthmatic who wanted to attend.

part
three

The Failsafe Diet

17 Which foods affect your asthma?

Summary

Most asthmatics react only to one or two food chemicals. The question is, which ones?

- If you have ever noticed asthma after wine, pickled onions, dried apricots or sausages, then you can be fairly sure sulphites are a problem.
- If you have ever had asthma after a Chinese meal then MSG probably affects you.
- If aspirin has ever made your asthma worse, you are probably sensitive to salicylates.

If you have never noticed a reaction, you may still be unknowingly affected by one or more food chemicals.

For people with mild occasional asthma

If you have asthma only a few times a year, you might be able to work it out by keeping a diary of foods, medications and symptoms for you or your child. For each episode of asthma, read back over the last two days, and check for sulphites (p. 187) and other additives in foods and medications.

You might be able to pinpoint the problem from your diary. It is sometimes enough to reduce consumption of one particular additive, for example, switching from white wine to red wine which is lower in sulphites, especially during high-risk situations such as colds and flu or during the pollen season.

If your asthma started recently with the introduction of a new food, you might also be able to identify your problem. For some people, like the woman on p. 38, the answer can be as simple as switching from diet cola to regular cola. If this is not sufficient, read on.

Removing the guesswork

The very best way to pinpoint exactly what is causing your problem—and to become an expert about just what is in our foods—is to do the failsafe diet with challenges. This will remove the guesswork. Then you will know exactly which foods to be careful with, and you will be much better at identifying the contents of our foods. It is only four weeks out of your life, or 0.001 per cent of your time here on earth. Of course your life could be a lot shorter if you don't get your asthma under control.

> Our little girl (four and a half) is happier and healthier since beginning the elimination diet. She has had no asthma, croup or colds, so no midnight trips to the emergency department of the children's hospital for us in five months.

The hardest part about doing an elimination diet is making the decision to start. Follow the checklist in the next section (p. 160). If you have more problems than just asthma, you might as well do an elimination diet to find out how good you and your family can feel. If there is no history of food intolerance and your asthma is only mild, you might like to do only the additive-free part of the diet.

Additive-free eating

Going additive-free is much more difficult than it sounds. Mothers often say to me, 'but we don't eat additives'. What they mean is that they don't eat takeaways. When I look at what they do eat, I often find 25 or more doses of additives per day in their 'healthy' food. A homemade cheese sandwich can contain five harmful additives—preservative in bread, colour and preservative in margarine, and colour and preservative in a slice of cheese. Add one or two more preservatives for a slice of ham or devon. Wash it down with a glass of fruit flavoured drink—'but it's very diluted', they say—and you can add two more each of colours and preservatives. That's a total of 11 harmful additives just for lunch, including sulphites.

Or you might choose a 'healthy' fruit bar for a snack. A health food apple and yoghurt snack lists natural colours and sulphites (220) but a call to the company reveals that the 'natural colours' are really artificial colours tartrazine (102) and sunset yellow (110). You are better off eating an apple.

The best way to go additive-free is to do the elimination diet as described in the lists and recipes in this book, but also allow yourself fresh home-prepared natural fruit (except grapes) and vegetables—not dried, processed, juiced, cooked or preprepared in any way. Think of it as a four week hands-on course about food additives. You will learn a lot and as a bonus, you will find out what contributes to your asthma. If asthma is still a problem

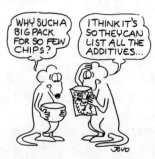

you may need to do the elimination diet again, this time fully failsafe and dairy free.

If you are pregnant: you can reduce your baby's risk of asthma by breastfeeding exclusively for at least four months. Eating Lactobacillus GG and avoiding antibiotics can help (see p. 119). Allergies run in families. If there are allergies on either side of the family, you might like to avoid peanuts and peanut products (see p. 208) from the last six weeks of pregnancy through breastfeeding, as well as egg or milk if those are family problems. Delay introduction of those foods until baby is one year old. Since food additives pass through breastmilk, if there is a family history of food intolerance you might like to go additive-free while breastfeeding. It is not only possible to do the failsafe diet while breastfeeding, this is considered a good time, while you still have total control over baby's diet. Of course, you will need to be supervised by a failsafe-friendly dietitian.

If you are a doctor: patients who would like to investigate dietary management of asthma can be referred to a dietitian experienced in supervising the Royal Prince Alfred Hospital elimination diet (see p. 300).

If diet is not enough: there are suggestions that the rebound effect of some drugs can make it difficult to stop taking your medication. If you have this problem, try a breathing technique (see p. 147). This can reduce your need for medication but does not seem to improve lung function, so do the diet as well.

Always carry a puffer: no matter how long you have gone without asthma, always carry a puffer with you for emergencies—yours and other people's.

Know your asthma first aid: see p. 114.

What's your food intolerance score?

It's important to rate your child or yourself on food intolerance reactions so that you have a baseline from which to measure your progress, instead of having to rely on your memory. Keep a record of your score before you start the elimination diet, and at intervals, for instance, after four weeks and after challenges.

Mark how much each symptom bothers you, where 0 is not at all and 3 is very much

SYMPTOM	SCORE			
Airways				
Asthma	0	1	2	3
Emphysema	0	1	2	3
Stuffy or runny nose	0	1	2	3
Frequent nose bleeds	0	1	2	3
Catarrh or chronic throat-clearing	0	1	2	3
Sinusitis	0	1	2	3
Frequent ear infections	0	1	2	3
Frequent tonsillitis	0	1	2	3
Frequent colds and flu	0	1	2	3
Skin				
Eczema	0	1	2	3
Urticaria (hives)	0	1	2	3
Other skin rashes	0	1	2	3
Angioedema (swollen lips, eyes, tongue)	0	1	2	3
Geographic tongue	0	1	2	3
Pruritis (itching)	0	1	2	3
Allergic shiners (dark circles under eyes)	0	1	2	3
Pallor (pale skin)	0	1	2	3
Flushing	0	1	2	3
Sweating	0	1	2	3
Body odour	0	1	2	3
Digestive system				
Recurrent mouth ulcers	0	1	2	3
Indigestion	0	1	2	3
Nausea	0	1	2	3
Bad breath	0	1	2	3
Vomiting	0	1	2	3
Diarrhoea	0	1	2	3
Stomach ache	0	1	2	3
Bloating	0	1	2	3
Reflux	0	1	2	3
Colic in babies	0	1	2	3
Sluggish bowel syndrome (sticky poos)	0	1	2	3
Soiling (sneaky poos)	0	1	2	3

Bladder

Bedwetting	0	1	2	3
Daytime incontinence	0	1	2	3
Urinary urgency	0	1	2	3
Recurrent inflammation (cystitis)	0	1	2	3

Skeletal

'Growing pains'	0	1	2	3
Arthritis	0	1	2	3

Eyes

Nystagmus (involuntary movement)	0	1	2	3
Blurred vision	0	1	2	3

Muscles

Low muscle tone	0	1	2	3
Myalgia (muscle pain)	0	1	2	3
Tics (involuntary movement)	0	1	2	3
Tremor	0	1	2	3
Palpitations	0	1	2	3
Tachycardia (fast heart beat)	0	1	2	3
Angina-type pain	0	1	2	3

Central nervous system

Headaches or migraines	0	1	2	3
Unexplained tiredness	0	1	2	3
Feeling 'hung-over'	0	1	2	3
Confusion	0	1	2	3
Dizziness	0	1	2	3
Agitation	0	1	2	3
Tinnitus (noises in ear)	0	1	2	3
Paraesthesia (pins and needles)	0	1	2	3
Dysaesthesia (numbness)	0	1	2	3
Epileptic seizures	0	1	2	3

Anxiety

Anxiety	0	1	2	3
Panic attacks	0	1	2	3
Depression	0	1	2	3
Suicidal thoughts, actions	0	1	2	3

Impaired memory   0   1   2   3
Vague or forgetful   0   1   2   3
Unable to concentrate   0   1   2   3
Won't persevere   0   1   2   3
Unmotivated   0   1   2   3
Disorganised   0   1   2   3
Easily distracted   0   1   2   3
Difficulty reading and writing 0   1   2   3

Speech
Loud voice (no volume control) 0   1   2   3
Speech hard to understand   0   1   2   3
Speech delay   0   1   2   3
Repetitive noises   0   1   2   3
Talks too much (empty chatter) 0   1   2   3

Coordination
Poor handwriting   0   1   2   3
Poor coordination   0   1   2   3
Frequent accidents   0   1   2   3

Sleep
Difficulty falling asleep   0   1   2   3
Restless legs   0   1   2   3
Persistent night waking   0   1   2   3
Insomnia   0   1   2   3
Nightmares/night terrors   0   1   2   3

Mood
Mood swings   0   1   2   3
Premenstrual tension   0   1   2   3
Grizzly or unhappy   0   1   2   3
Cries easily or often   0   1   2   3
Irritable   0   1   2   3
Uncooperative   0   1   2   3

Oppositional defiance
Loses temper   0   1   2   3
Argumentative   0   1   2   3
Refuses requests   0   1   2   3
Defies rules   0   1   2   3
Deliberately annoys others   0   1   2   3
Blames others for own mistakes 0   1   2   3

Touchy, easily annoyed	0	1	2	3
Angry, resentful	0	1	2	3

Other behaviour

Inattentive, easily bored, unmotivated	0	1	2	3
Restless, fidgety or overactive	0	1	2	3
Head banging	0	1	2	3
Fights with siblings	0	1	2	3
Difficulty making friends	0	1	2	3
Destructive, aggressive	0	1	2	3
Unreasonable	0	1	2	3
Demanding, never satisfied	0	1	2	3
Disruptive	0	1	2	3
Discipline is ineffective	0	1	2	3

Total

Remember, write down your score before and after the elimination diet so you can see the difference.

18 How to start the Failsafe Diet

A step-by-step guide

1. **Check with your doctor** that your problem really is asthma. If you suspect allergies, you can ask for skin prick tests.

2. **Find a failsafe friendly dietitian** by asking hospital, community or private dietitians (look in the Yellow Pages) if they have experience in supervising the elimination diet from Royal Prince Alfred Hospital, or contact the Food Intolerance Network (p. 299).

3. **If weight loss is a problem** especially for children, weigh your child and record the weight once a week. If a skinny child loses weight, ask your dietitian about caloric supplements such as Polycose or stop the diet.

4. **Decide how many foods** you will exclude. This is the hard part. If you don't exclude enough food chemicals, the diet won't work. If you want to avoid *additives but not salicylates* see p. 187. For chronic asthma, the best place to start is *failsafe* (free of additives, low in salicylates, amines and flavour enhancers). This is the diet outlined on p. 219. If you have any reason at all to suspect *dairy foods*—you have seen a reaction, there is a history of milk allergy, you or your child has a pale face, dark circles under eyes, your child had lactose intolerance as a baby, frequent ear infections, grommets, would live on milk if you let him/her, drinks litres of milk a day, or hates milk—avoid all dairy products (see p. 206). For severe problems you might need to avoid *wheat or gluten* as well. A family history of irritable bowel or especially a family member with coeliac disease is an indication of possible problems (see p. 209).

5. **Read the failsafe diet lists** on pages 219–231 and shopping list on pages 232–239.

6. **Check product updates** on the web (www.fedupwith foodadditives.info) in case manufacturers have changed ingredients.

7. **Establish a failsafe house** by eating or giving away all the unsuitable food in your kitchen. It is best if at least one other family member does the diet and the whole family must appear to do this diet at home. Children who are expected to stick to this diet while others at home eat tempting foods will very reasonably sneak food or money.

8. **Negotiate incentives with your child** ('what's this worth to you?'). A daily reward with a bonus after three weeks is better than one big bribe. Ask for the support of your partner and anyone else in the household.

9. **Mark D-day**—diet day—on your calendar, preferably on a Monday. You might want to wait until a special occasion, birthday party or school camp is out of the way.

10. Using the recipes, **draw up a week's menu plan**, including snacks, which you feel is workable for your family. It doesn't have to include a lot of variety. In the first three weeks, you just want to get rid of food chemicals and cravings.

11. **Go shopping**. Take a list of the ingredients you need for your recipes and the shopping list on pages 232–39 for other ideas. Also take the *Additives to Avoid* card included with this book with you. The first failsafe shop will be time consuming while you read labels, after that it will be quicker and cheaper than usual.

12. **Try out some recipes** before you get to D-day. For children, cook and freeze some meals and treats like failsafe

mince (p. 248), cakes and biscuits. Have magic cordial (p. 246), pear jam (p. 256) and icypoles (p. 246) ready.

13. **Rate symptoms** on the food intolerance score sheet on pages 000–00 so that you have a baseline from which to measure your progress.

14. On D-day, **start the diet**. Keep taking your asthma medication.

15. Doing this diet alone can be difficult. If you don't have a failsafe friend, **supports** are available through the Food Intolerance Network. Consider joining an email failsafe discussion group (p. 299). It is worth joining the free email newsletter list for product updates and recipes.

16. **Keep a diary** of everything that goes in the mouth or on the skin (foods, toothpaste, medications). Record peak flow readings two or three times a day and any other symptom— health, behaviour, learning—during the diet. It is easier to see effects when looking back.

17. **Expect withdrawal symptoms** within the first two weeks, often on days four and five. These can include tearfulness, food cravings and irritability as well as whatever your reason is for doing the diet—such as irritable airways, croup (see p. 167) or over-the-top behaviour. You might like to try an antidote (p. 179). Take asthma medication as required. You can minimise withdrawals by reducing additive intake over a few weeks—and don't binge on takeaways the weekend before starting the diet.

18. **Read the checklist of common mistakes** (p. 273) many times. If there is no improvement after two weeks, ask your dietitian or support group for help.

19. **Rate your progress** after three to six weeks (for behaviour, three weeks is usually enough, asthma and skin rashes may take longer).

20. You are ready to **start challenges** (p. 167) when you have five good days in a row after three to six weeks. Asthmatics *must* have challenges supervised by a dietitian.

21. If you are doing the diet with a difficult child, as your child becomes more amenable to discipline, **establish a**

behaviour management program in your household
(p. 300).

22. When you have learned which foods affect you and established a new food routine, go back to your dietitian and
have your nutrition checked if you are avoiding salicylates, dairy foods or gluten.

23. Food chemical sensitivity varies depending on the total load
to which we are exposed. Environmental chemicals, stress,
lack of sleep, illness and hormones can all contribute.
Avoid unnecessary chemicals (p. 218) and allow time for
exercise, sleep and relaxation.

24. Most children eat a fairly high-sugar, high-fat diet when
being weaned off processed foods. As your child's tastes
settle down, reduce the intake of fats and sugars, and **eat
more failsafe vegetables**.

Challenges

After three to six weeks of the elimination diet (p. 219), you
must test whether you are sensitive to salicylates and amines,
otherwise you may be restricting healthy foods unnecessarily.
If you are avoiding dairy foods, wheat or gluten, the same
applies. Exceptionally sensitive babies need not challenge
because reactions to small amounts of salicylate or amine-
containing foods will be obvious.

Challenges can be carried out with foods or capsules.
Teaching hospitals use capsule challenges, which give quick
and obvious results. Because capsule challenges involve a big
dose, asthmatics are routinely hospitalised for capsule challenges like sulphites, salicylates and MSG so that resuscitation
equipment is available. Food challenges are not as strong but
supervision is still required for asthmatics. Discuss this with
your dietitian or doctor.

A five-year-old suffered recurrent asthma associated with
croup about once a month from the age of four months until
she went failsafe. On the first night of both the sulphite and
benzoate challenges, she developed croup, followed by

asthma—as usual—four days later. On her doctor's suggestion, she used a puffer from the beginning of the croup.

The rules of challenge:
- **Five good days** in a row before the first challenge.
- **Three good days** in a row before subsequent challenges.
- **Stick strictly** to the elimination diet during challenges. Start again (three good days) if you make a mistake.
- **Do one challenge at a time** or you won't know which food chemical caused the reaction.

> A mother was doing the diet with her asthmatic son for behaviour. Since it was Easter, her dietitian agreed to an Easter egg challenge which is combined dairy and amines. 'I couldn't tell what his behaviour was like,' she said, 'because he ended up in hospital with his asthma.' She hadn't even realised that her son's asthma was related to food—'You're right, his asthma had gone away on the diet.'

- **Eat only specified foods.** Foods like oranges and tomatoes have no place in challenges because they contain more than one food chemical (salicylates *and* amines).
- **Take note of any symptoms from pages 160–63 which occur during the challenge.** For more subtle conditions you might have to set up a daily test like exercise for asthma or similar homework with your child to test poor concentration.
- **Eat enough challenge foods**, at least the minimum amount every day. If you start slowly, you may get confusing results.
- **Continue until you see a reaction**. Three days for additives except 282, otherwise a full seven days but ten days may be needed for the dairy challenge. For complicating factors such as illness, major stress (crashing your car) or unexpected chemical exposure (carpet cleaned, schoolroom painted), stop the challenge, wait for three good days and start again.

- **Stop when you see a reaction.** You can then use an antidote.
- **No mini challenges**. Do not conclude that 'he reacts to orange juice but he's OK with apricots'. That's not the way it works. Every food which contains salicylates—like apricots—will contribute to occasional obvious reactions or good days and bad days with no obvious cause. The same goes for amines and 'she's OK with bananas but can't handle chocolate'.

First challenge

Do challenges in any order you want. In theory, you should be able to add back into your diet any group of food chemicals that don't cause a reaction. However, in practice, people make a lot of mistakes when doing this—such as thinking 'I don't react to salicylates so I can eat broccoli again' although broccoli contains both salicylates and amines—so it is better to finish all your challenges before adding back food chemicals you can tolerate.

SALICYLATE CHALLENGE

Eat at least six serves every day for seven to ten days of the following foods. Stop when you see a reaction. One serve equals approximately one cup of mango, asparagus, carrot, pumpkin, capsicum, corn, cucumber, zucchini, Granny Smith apple, apricots, peaches, nectarines, cherries, strawberries, rockmelons or watermelons. Use also 1 tsp cinnamon or curry-type spices (turmeric, cardamom, coriander, cumin, garam marsala, ginger, paprika, pepper) in powder form (not paste), 1 tbsp honey, 150 ml of preservative-free apple juice, 1 cup strong tea or peppermint tea. Use moderate salicylate options in recipes. None of the very high salicylate foods (tomatoes, oranges, sultanas, pineapple, grapes) are suitable for the challenge because they all contain amines as well.

AMINE CHALLENGE

Eat two to three ripe bananas and 60–120 g dark chocolate (half for small children) until there is an obvious reaction or for at least seven days. Amine reactions are usually delayed up to several days or more. For dark chocolate use Nestle dark chocolate choc bits, Old Gold, Jamaica, or cooking chocolate.

For children who don't like dark chocolate—although most do after three weeks on the elimination diet—you can cook the choc bits into chocolate cake or banana muffins, or freeze the bananas and process into banana icecream topped with melted chocolate. Eat also as much as you want of: canned tuna, salmon, sardines, frozen fish, pork chops and roast pork (but not bacon and ham).

If you react to both salicylates and amines, once you are convinced there is a reaction, you can use an antidote (p. 179). People who react to both salicylates and amines can stop challenges now as they will probably react to additives as well.

SULPHITES (220–228)
Most foods which contain sulphites (e.g. wine, dried fruit and vegetables, and sausages) also contain salicylates or amines so it is best to do those challenges first. If you don't react to salicylates, you can challenge sulphites by eating seven dried apricot halves every day for three days.

BENZOATES (210–213)
Drink 1 litre of preserved lemonade (211) a day for three days.

MSG (621 AND NATURAL GLUTAMATES)
Mix 4 tbsp soy sauce into a meal, e.g. fried rice, every day for three days.

Vegetable haters who will eat green peas might challenge peas (small amounts of natural glutamates) early. For a **green pea challenge**, eat green peas twice a day every day for three days. If no reaction, you can add peas back into the diet. People who fail the MSG challenge can often manage green peas.

NITRATES (249–252)
Eat 4 slices of ham, bacon or corned beef per day. Not for amine reactors.

COLOUR CHALLENGE
Put 5 drops of green food colouring in water or magic cordial (p. 246) three times a day for one day followed by the same procedure with 10 drops of red and 10 drops of yellow.

ANTIOXIDANT CHALLENGE—GALLATES (310–312) AND TBHQ, BHA, BHT (319–321)
Some people react to the second group but not to the first. Use 3 tbsp of cooking oil or margarine containing one or the other group, every day for three days. You might like to use the cooking oil to deep fry home-cooked hot chips. For THBQ and BHA you can use Lay's plain potato chips.

DAIRY AND WHEAT CHALLENGES
These should be done at some stage if you are avoiding dairy (one to three cups of milk every day for ten days) and wheat (one cup of plain uncoloured cooked pasta plus 12 water crackers every day for seven days).

BREAD PRESERVATIVE (282)
Shopping is easier if you pass this challenge and so it is worth doing. Sometimes the label says bread contains preservative when it doesn't so it is safest to challenge with two crumpets, two English toasted muffins, or four slices of preserved bread during summer every day for a week.

ANNATTO COLOUR (160B)
This should be challenged especially if you can eat dairy products because it is in so many foods. Eat one tub of coloured yoghurt every day for three days. Some people react to only a few additives, yet if they eat them every day, then the result can be the same as for a person who reacts to everything.

FLAVOUR ENHANCER 635 (ALSO CALLED RIBONUCLEOTIDES)
If you don't react to salicylates, MSG or preservatives, eat one packet of Maggi instant chicken flavoured noodles or one packet of CC's corn chips every day for three days and have antihistamines handy.

SORBATES (200–203)
Eat 100 g of preserved cottage cheese and 1 tbsp of low fat spread containing 202.

SUGAR
This challenge is optional. It is for people who are convinced their children react to sugar with hyperactivity or hypoglycaemic symptoms. In nearly all cases, this will be due to salicylates or additives. However, there are a very few extremely sensitive people who do react to white sugar. You need to test this with a challenge. Eat ten sugar cubes in one day and observe reactions. If no reaction, double the amount and eat in one day.

OTHER CHALLENGES
You can choose to challenge anything you want, from favourite foods to herbal supplements. Just follow the rules. My children chose their favourite chocolate bar—every day for three days—and failed.

For more details see the RPAH booklet from your dietitian.

After challenges—testing tolerance
If you are sensitive to salicylates, you have two choices: you can find your tolerance and stay within the limits, or you can try to build tolerance by sticking to low salicylate foods for six months. When reintroducing salicylates, eat one moderate serve (carrots, corn or pumpkin) every second day for two weeks. If no reaction, increase to one serve every day for two weeks. If still OK, increase the dose to one cup every second day for two weeks and so on. Go back to the last level if you start reacting.

> I am at the stage now where I have reintroduced amines into my diet about twice a week, with the exception of my premenstrual week. I am prone to being overconfident and blowing my reintroduction from time-to-time but I have pretty much worked out the timing and culprits.
> —Reader, NSW

Frequently asked questions

Q. My 14 year old son gets asthma only during the pollen season. Does this mean his asthma is not related to foods?

A. No, it means that his asthma is not *triggered* by foods. For most people food chemicals are much more likely to cause irritable airways than to trigger an asthma attack. When these irritable airways are then exposed to a trigger—like pollen—asthma is the result. It could be that your son needs only to avoid, for example, sulphites during the pollen season.

Q. Is Nutella failsafe?

A. There are no additives in Nutella but it is is high in salicylates (hazelnuts) and amines (chocolate and hazelnuts). For people with nut allergies, Nutella is one of the top three hidden traps. The others are chocolate and muesli bars.

Q. My three year old gets growing pains in his legs. They're so bad they keep him awake. He cries from the pain.

A. It could be any food chemical, however, in my experience, growing pains are often associated with nitrates and nitrites (249–252) in processed meats like bacon, ham and devon. **Response:** 'Oh, my God! He loves devon, he just about lives on it!'

A. Devon also contains sodium metabisulphite, an asthma additive.

Q. At the daycare centre where I work, we gave a peanut butter sandwich to a nine-month-old baby. She had an immediate reaction to it and we have been told she must never have any form of peanut again or she could die. Did we cause her allergy?

A. Allergy is a combination of susceptibility and exposure. Peanut allergy usually becomes obvious the first time the child eats peanut butter, but the baby was probably already sensitised (see p. 208). Many schools and childcare centres in the US and increasingly in Australia have banned peanut butter.

Q. A woman who used to work on a prawn trawler told me the prawns were always sprinkled with metabisulphite powder to improve the colour. Do they still do this? How do people know if this has been done when they buy the prawns?

A. Prawns always contain added sulphites. Our national food regulators make the rules but the states are responsible for consumer education and enforcement. Apparently they assume that people who are sensitive to sulphites will recognise their sensitivity and will read the FSANZ leaflet called 'Are sulphites safe?' The answer is essentially that sulphites are not safe for sulphite-sensitive asthmatics. The leaflet advises asthmatics to avoid prawns and other foods which contain sulphites (see list p. 188–89) and to carry an asthma inhaler at all times.

Q. Are fish oil supplements failsafe?

A. All fish oil supplements contain amines and Efalex also contains salicylates in thyme oil, so they are not failsafe. There is evidence that the omega-3 fatty acids in fish oils help to prevent inflammation, which is why Sydney researchers are currently testing the effects of fish oils on asthmatic children. They are aiming for an omega-3 to omega-6 fatty acid ratio of roughly 1:5 (compared to 1:15 in the general population) through the use of tuna fish oil supplements plus canola based oils and margarines. Canola is failsafe and very fresh white fish is failsafe. If you want to use fish oils, pass your amine challenge first, or test them according to the rules of challenge, p. 168.

Q. I bought a muesli bar which listed natural colour but didn't say which one. When I phoned I found it was actually two artificial colours (tartrazine 102 and sunset yellow 110). What should I do?

A. There isn't much you can do other than complain to your local council or health department (it varies in each state). Of 13 complaints I have submitted only two were addressed. For mislabelling, the company will usually say they are using up old packaging. In the unlikely event of prosecution, the fines are ridiculously small. However, if more consumers lodged complaints, the problem cannot be ignored.

Q. Help! I'd like to try the diet but I don't know where to start.
A. See p. 164 for step-by-step instructions, and this mother's experience might help you: 'I think the biggest hurdle is that first shopping trip. I picked out several recipes I wanted to try, and carefully reviewed the list of acceptable foods. I made sure I put all the ingredients I needed for the recipes on my shopping list, along with acceptable foods, including goodies like chips and ice cream. At the supermarket it did take a long time to find all the new things I was buying, but when I got home, I had a kitchen full of failsafe products and all the ingredients I needed for some failsafe recipes.'

Q. You say that failsafers get fewer colds, flu and other infections. How can that happen?
A. Studies suggest that nitrite and propionate preservatives and possibly some artificial colours have an immunosuppressant effect, that is, they stop the immune system from preventing infections. This is reversible when exposure to the food chemical stops. Presumably some people are more vulnerable to this effect than others and some other food chemicals have the same effect.

Q. Isn't this diet very high in sugar? I am worried about my children's teeth.
A. Tooth decay was a big topic in one of the email discussion groups. We had all noticed that our children's teeth have been much better since we switched to failsafe—which was the opposite of what we expected. Perhaps it is because failsafe children no longer consume fruit juice and dried fruit which are known problems for teeth. Or it could be that this diet appears to be high in sugar but is actually very low in hidden sugars in processed foods such as 10 tsp of sugar per can of soft drink.

Q. What about nutrition?
A. If you eat a wide range of permitted foods and take recommended supplements, failsafe is nutritionally adequate, but it can be low in Vitamin A and Vitamin C if you don't eat permitted vegetables; low in calcium if you don't have dairy foods or calcium-fortified substitutes; and low in protein and B group Vitamins if you are wheat- or gluten-free. In the short term, take permitted multivitamin supplements every day (see p. 239). In the long term, work towards eating more vegetables (see below), take calcium supplements if needed, and eat more meat or dried beans if gluten-free. Have your family's nutrition checked by your dietitian when you have done your challenges and have become established on the diet. When expanding or breaking the diet—and everyone does sometimes—choose nutritious fruit and vegetables from the moderate column like mango, corn or carrots but don't overdo it or you will be back where you started.

Q. My son won't eat *any* failsafe vegetables. He only eats broccoli and tomatoes.
A. Tastes do change. Or you can try the failsafe soup trick. It goes like this. Buy a lot of small toys as rewards. Try bland failsafe vegetables like potato, leek and cabbage with a bit of salt, thoroughly blended. Get him to put a tiny amount on a teaspoon in his mouth the first night (doesn't matter if he eats it or not) for a reward. The next night make it a small lick for a reward, then double it each night. After two weeks he should be eating a cup of vegetable soup every night. Stop the rewards and start hiding other vegetables, even Brussels sprouts. Or see Mum's mash, p. 251.

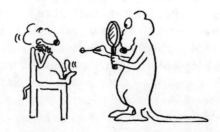

Q. Isn't the failsafe diet difficult socially?
A. Yes, it is, and this is the major disadvantage of going failsafe. Everyone says, 'Eating at home is easy, eating out is a problem.' But do you really want to feed your family food which makes them ill? For more about the economics, politics and ethics of processed food, see *Fast Food Nation* (p. 300). I prefer to defy peer pressure by buying food which makes my family healthy and happy. Since a growing number of us feel the same way, you can choose to socialise with other failsafers.

Q. You mention that exposure to certain toxic chemicals can make people more sensitive to other chemicals. Can you say what some of these 'sensitisers' are?
A. I doubt this is a complete list: gasoline (petrol), kerosene, natural gas, pesticides (especially chlordane and chlorpyrifos), solvents, new carpet and other renovation materials, adhesives/glues, fibreglass, carbonless copy paper, fabric softener, formaldehyde and glutaraldehyde, carpet shampoos (lauryl sulfate) and other cleaning agents, isocyanates, combustion products (poorly vented gas heaters, overheated batteries), and medications (prolonged antibiotics, general anaesthesia with petrochemicals, intranasally packed neosynephrine, and dinitrichlorobenzene for warts). Repeated low-level exposure may be as harmful as a single, acute exposure.

Q. My daughter has been on the elimination diet for two weeks now and is tired of the plain meals as she calls them.
A. At the end of the second week there is a flat patch where withdrawal symptoms have finished, the novelty has worn off and the food seems boring, the end of the third week seems like a long way away and everyone says, 'Well, I think there is an improvement but it might be due to something else.' It will pass. You might like to buy a new toy or video as a distraction or cook something special from the desserts section—'Would you like Lemon meringue pie in your lunchbox today?' If you have already seen any improvement, then you should see continuing small improvements until you will realise—at about the end of

the third or fourth week (unless you are making a mistake)—
that it really was worthwhile after all.

**Q. Last night my son had a really bad bout of croup. We
have just started our elimination diet and he has been doing
so well. Our GP said another night like last night means
he needs to be on prednisolone or steroids. She thinks it is
flavoured and will have preservatives in it.**

A. Steroid syrup for children contains benzoates and raspberry
flavour so it is not failsafe. You could ask for white tablets
instead, but there are suggestions that steroids themselves have
potential side effects including aggressive behaviour, anxiety
and hyperactivity. For children with uncontrollable outbursts
that may be caused by food or drug chemicals, stay calm, avoid
confrontations and use a cooperative approach (see *The Explosive Child*, p. 300). Introduce some moderate salicylates to
reduce the boredom. Resume the diet when you have finished
the medication. Don't despair. In the long term, failsafe kids
stop getting croup and other illnesses.

Q. How safe are soy products?
A. There is a lot of controversy surrounding soy. You will have
to decide this one for yourself. The most balanced and scientific
article I have seen is available on the web at Harvard Women's
Health Watch, (www.health.harvard.edu/medline/Women/
W801a.html). I still drink soymilk in moderation.

Q. Isn't the diet too hard?
A. It is much harder than it needs to be because the food
industry has forced us to accept widespread use of potentially
harmful additives in our most basic foods. There are two ways
you can deal with this. You can take medication to deal with the
side effects of your food or you can *refuse to buy* foods containing harmful additives. If we all did that, food manufacturers
would change their ingredients very quickly! For people who
decide on option two, joining the newsletter list and an email
discussion group or support group will make you feel much less
isolated (see p. 299).

Mothers complained about the difficulties of eating out, kids' parties, spending so long in the kitchen, the feelings of guilt in denying their children their favourite foods, and the stress of having to say no all the time (pretty much what the email group discusses) . . . It is such a shame that it is not easier to 'do the diet'—that there is so much food that we can't buy, just because of unnecessary ingredients.—*Member of email discussion group*

Q. Salicylates don't seem to affect us too badly. I think we can manage moderates and some high-salicylate fruit and vegetables.
A. Be careful. You will *never* see a reaction to a few salicylate-containing foods. There is always a build up which is difficult to detect. Beware of outsiders who say 'but an apple/piece of fruit a day won't hurt you'. You won't notice any reaction at first, so you will think you are not so sensitive. The effects of salicylates can build up slowly and eventually you will be back where you started. If you are worried about nutrition, eat permitted vegetables and take permitted vitamin and mineral supplements (see shopping list p. 232). A few people are extremely sensitive to salicylates (see checklist of common mistakes, p. 273).

Q. What if we make a mistake?
A. Here is an **antidote for food reactions**: we used to call this SOS powder. It is an old home remedy for food intolerance. The effects last for about an hour.

2 parts bicarbonate of soda
1 part calcium carbonate
1 part potassium bicarbonate

The recommended dose is 1 tsp or less, three times per day, in a glass of water or diluted in magic cordial (p. 246), until the condition settles. For small children, just a pinch of powder can be enough to help. If you can't get all those ingredients from your pharmacist, you can make do with half a tsp of bicarbonate of soda or less (soda bicarb from your pantry) in the same way. Or a calcium carbonate calcium supplement (see p. 239). These antidotes work for reflux, stomach aches, headaches, skin rashes, restless legs, insomnia, irritability and hyperactivity. Do they work for asthma? I don't know. You should have a puffer handy at all times.

Q. Why hasn't my doctor told me about the diet?
A. Pressure from vested interests—the pharmaceutical industry and food industry—is immense. Doctors are one of the main targets. Most do not realise how they have been pressured (see p. 80). The study of medicine has become essentially the study of medications and non-profit making therapies are ignored. Doctors should be in the front line protecting our children from harmful chemicals in their food and environment, but a lot aren't. There are some exceptions like the wonderful doctors at the Centre for Children's Health and the Environment (www.childenvironment.org), Greater Boston Physicians for Social Responsibility (www.igc.org/psr/) and those who support the Center for Science in the Public Interest (www.cspinet.org).

Q. How can I get a difficult child to stick to this diet?
A. Failsafe your house. Eat, give away or throw out unsuitable foods. It doesn't work to have a fridge full of cola and chocolates and say 'you can't have those'. Everyone in the house must appear to do the diet too—they can eat what they want when outside. It is best for the mother to do the diet with the child, as a role model. Younger children should also follow the diet or they will brag when you're not around.

Praise and reward. Tell the child often how good he is for sticking to the diet and how much you admire him. At the end of every day give a small reward for sticking to the diet. This can be stickers or tokens towards a larger reward.

You must be able to say no to your child, as in 'no, you can't have that food right now, but how would you like something else?'. The video *1–2–3 Magic* is fun to watch and it works. Or try a parenting class like Triple P (p. 301).

Avoid brainwashing in the form of television advertising. In 1995, the American Academy of Pediatrics announced that 'advertising directed at children is inherently deceptive and exploits children under eight years of age'. Not only that, one study found that 95 per cent of advertisements during children's prime time were advertising junk food. Turn off the TV and watch videos instead. If you have to watch your favourite show, tape it and fast forward through the ads.

Join an email discussion group, support group or failsafe playgroup so that you don't feel alone (p. 299).

Q. I hate cooking.
A. So do I. The way I manage is by being organised. I choose very simple meals and have a weekly plan (p. 240). My husband and children share the load of cooking, cleaning up and shopping.

Q. My family says the food is too bland.
A. The food industry has worked very hard to make you a flavour junkie. But tastes do change. After a few months you can really enjoy the flavour of very fresh, natural food again and it is common for failsafe kids to enthuse over the taste of a carrot. In the meantime, you can use unlimited garlic and it is OK to add salt, because this diet is very low in processed foods with hidden salt. Buy quality ingredients. Fresh fish, lamb steak and real maple syrup may seem expensive but they are a lot cheaper than eating out. If you enjoy cooking, have the time, and want gourmet foods for adults, try the Royal Prince Alfred Hospital Allergy Clinic's recipe book *Friendly Food* (see p. 300). It is not usually a success with children.

Q. Any hints about eating out?
A. It is best to find a restaurant which suits you and go there often. Eating out in a new place is always a risk. One high-powered career woman who has to eat out frequently and is very food sensitive phones the chef beforehand and orders steamed white fresh fish, steamed white rice (no flavours) and steamed green beans. She drinks soda water and she never has any

problems. I'm not as organised as that. I eat before I go so I'm not too hungry, and order plain foods like steak and jacket potato or fish with no sauce. Natural oysters are failsafe. If the restaurant bakes its own bread, it might be preservative-free bread. An easy way to enjoy the company of friends in a café is to eat before you go and have a decaf coffee. For fast food, see next question. If sulphites are your only problem, see p. 187.

Q. What's the safest takeaway food?
A. I used to recommend plain rotisseried chicken but it is no longer possible to buy BBQ chicken without seasoned skin. Try jacket baked potato from a potato cart. The slimmers' special (cottage cheese and chives) is one of the best but contains sorbates and dairy foods. You can take your own Nuttelex spread. One mother asks a local Chinese café to prepare fried rice consisting only of rice, shallots and egg. This is enough to give the family a cooking-free Friday night. We usually choose grilled fish—although not in Darwin where it has all been frozen—but this is unsuitable if you react to amines. Ask for the freshest white fish. Grilled is best because it avoids colours in the crumbs or batter and antioxidants like BHA (320) or TBHQ (319) in the oil. Avoid chips or fries because of antioxidants in the oil and sulphites in the chips. Take your own fresh buttered preservative-free bread rolls with lettuce and make fish burgers. See p. 191 for other suggestions—you will have to test it for yourself, but not during your strict elimination diet.

Q. I have a question about a food not on the list.
A. If the food isn't on the list, apply the taste test. Assume all fruit except pears contain some salicylates, the stronger the flavour, the more salicylates. If you like it, you can't have it. For meats, the stronger the flavour, the higher the amines. You can do a careful challenge. Stick to the rules (see p. 168). Don't just eat it once and assume it is OK.

Q. Are there any failsafe ways of dealing with constipation?
A. First, distinguish between true constipation (hard, dry

stools, sometimes like 'rabbit pellets', due to lack of liquids and fibre) and sluggish bowel due to food intolerance which can resemble constipation. With sluggish bowel, there is a feeling of incomplete evacuation ('always more to come'). Faeces are sticky and hard to clean up. For true constipation, drink lots of water or magic cordial (p. 246, sugar has a mild laxative effect), eat more fibre found in pears, celery, cabbage, other vegetables especially beans and lentils, rhubarb (moderate in salicylates but good for constipation), rolled oats, All Bran, rice bran, and oily foods like fries—home-made, of course. For sluggish bowel, use rice bran or psyllium hulls (be careful if atopic, some people are allergic to these) when needed, but it is important to identify and avoid your problem food chemicals. If salicylate-sensitive, the worst thing you can do is eat high salicylate fruit and especially prune juice, because salicylates often provoke this condition.

Q. We are happy to avoid additives but I can't see how it can be healthy to cut out fruit and vegetables.
A. For people who react to salicylates, most fruit and some vegetables are not healthy. This may be because the fruit and vegetables we eat now are very different from those eaten 100 years ago or it may be that exposure to toxic chemicals like pesticides has made us more sensitive to salicylates which are natural pesticides. It is only by avoiding salicylates that you can find out whether you are affected. It is possible to eat the recommended two serves a day of failsafe fruit and five serves a day of failsafe vegetables, which according to diet surveys is a lot more than the average child and especially teenager eats. Given a chance to find out how good they can feel without salicylates, many people say, 'Nothing will make me go back to the foods I previously loved so much.'

Q. I presume natural flavours are better than artificial flavours?
A. No, there's not much difference (see p. 206).

Q. What is the difference between vanilla and vanillin?
A. Vanilla is natural and vanillin is artificial. Vanilla is failsafe but only to the limit of two drops per day. Failsafe products which contain vanilla or vanillin may be OK if the taste is not too strong but it is a matter of dose. For example, a few Werther's original butter candies might be tolerated but a whole packet might be too much.

Q. How do we know which added flavours are failsafe?
A. Fruit flavours are not failsafe because of salicylates. Flavours in tasty foods are likely to contain glutamates (620–625) or ribonucleotides (627, 631, 635) often added but not declared on the label, so they are not failsafe. Strong flavours are often a problem. There are many reports of reactions to flavours in chocolate. Approach any product containing flavours with caution. Just because a small dose is OK, don't assume you can eat large quantities. As with other additives, effects are cumulative. During your elimination diet, avoid commercial products containing flavours unless they are included in the shopping list and even then, be careful.

Q. What about organic food?
A. As well as avoiding pesticide use inside and outside your home, the Center for Children's Health and the Environment recommends 'a wise diet' for children. This includes staying away from food additives and eating organic food. It is now thought that frequent low exposure to pesticides in early childhood may contribute to a range of conditions including asthma. Organic dairy foods are strongly recommended in the US, where bovine growth hormone is permitted. Organic meats and chickens are failsafe. However, organic food may not overcome the problem of sensitivity to natural food chemicals. If you can't eat an orange because of salicylates, then you probably can't eat an organic orange either. Organic fruit and vegetables which taste noticeably better than their non-organic counterparts are likely to be higher in salicylates.

Q. Is A2 milk safer for asthmatics?

A. Most Western breeds of dairy cattle produce milks that have a combination of A1 and A2 types of milk proteins. Research findings worldwide suggest that when beta casein A1 is broken down during digestion, it gives rise to beta-casamorphin-7 which has been linked with type 1 diabetes, heart disease, autism and schizophrenia. Goats, buffalo, yaks and African and Asian cows produce only A2 milk proteins. In New Zealand, the A2 Corporation produces A2 mild for consumers. Does this have any implications for asthmatics? We don't know yet. More details from www.a2corporation.com.

19 How to avoid problem foods

Read this chapter when you have completed your challenges and discovered which food chemicals you need to avoid. Don't be alarmed: you won't have to give up chicken and chips, hamburgers, pizza, fish and chips, stir-fries, spaghetti, icecream, cakes, alcohol or sugar—you just need to choose your food carefully, or cook it yourself. If enough people refuse to buy foods with additives, the food industry will provide more additive-free alternatives and staying healthy will be much easier.

How to avoid sulphites

For starters, avoid everything in the range 220–228, but many of the sulphites you eat will be in unlabelled foods.

220	Sulphur dioxide
221	Sodium sulphite
222	Sodium bisulphite
223	Sodium metabisulphite
224	Potassium metabisulphite
225	Potassium sulphite
228	Potassium bisulphite

When you look at the sulphite lists pp. 188–89, you can see why the failsafe diet works so well for sulphite-sensitive asthmatics. By avoiding processed foods and salicylates in fruit, fruit drinks, dried fruit, fruit flavoured breakfasts, cookies, snacks, muesli bars, yoghurt, icecream and confectionery, you are also getting rid of sulphites.

There is a big gap between reading sulphite lists and understanding whether the food you buy or a dish you order in a restaurant contains sulphites. Liz from p. 22 recommends: avoid sausages, all processed deli meat, cordials, jams, shop produced fruit salad, pickled anything with vinegar, shop bought hot chips, dried foods like apricots and 'anything that isn't natural'.

Although there are differences between Australia and the US, the sulphite lists on p. 190 give an idea of the size of the problem. 'Current regulations discourage the use of large amounts of sulfites,' says Rick Williams of the Nosulfites website. 'Today, the problem is low levels of sulfur dioxide in practically everything you touch.' Sulphites under 10 parts per million (ppm) do not have to be listed but they will all contribute to your sulphite intake. A survey in Australia found sulphites in more than half the foods tested including such staples as bread and margarine, with sulphites higher in white bread than wholemeal.

If you look at ingredient listings of fast food companies you will see that few of the ingredients have sulphites listed.

This does not mean that the foods are sulphite-free. There are small amounts of sulphites in processed food ingredients like corn syrup solids, cornstarch, maltodextrin, potato starch and flakes, beet sugar, bottled lemon juice used for flavouring and dressings, glucose syrup, the caramel colour used in cola drinks, and sulphites in pizza crust. They all add up.

The easiest way to avoid sulphites is to avoid all processed foods. The foods in the shopping list on p. 232 are sulphite-free. Fresh fruit and vegetables are supposed to be sulphite-free except for grapes. In Australia, dates, prunes, raisins and sultanas are the only dried fruit which have no sulphites listed on the label. You have to think about the ingredients in everything you eat. However, if you have done your elimination diet and challenges, and found that you react to only sulphites, then you can add back the food chemicals which don't cause problems. This is the hard part—reintroducing foods without making mistakes. If you start getting asthma again, you need to go back a few steps.

Sulphites in Australian foods

	Maximum permitted (ppm)
Alcoholic beverages	
Wine, sparkling and fortified, more than 35 g/L sugar	400
Wine as above, less than 35 g/L sugar	250
Wine (fruit, veg, mead), more than 5 g/L sugar	300
Wine as above, less than 5 g/L sugar	200
Mixed alcoholic drinks	250
Beer	25
Baked goods	
As a dough conditioner	60
Flour products incl. noodles and pasta	300
Biscuits, cakes and pastry	300
Beverages, non-alcoholic	
Fruit juice, drinks, soft drinks, cordials	115
Condiments and relishes	
Chutneys	285
Pickles, pickled onions, gherkins	750

Sulphites in Australian foods	Maximum permitted (ppm)
Vinegars and related products	100
Sauces and toppings, mayonnaise	350
Fish and shellfish	
Uncooked crustaceans (prawns, shrimps, crab, crayfish, lobster)	100
Cooked crustaceans	30
Fully preserved fish incl. canned products	30
Canned abalone	1000
Fresh fruit and vegetables	
Fresh prepared salads and fruit salads	illegal but it happens
Grapes packed with permeable envelopes	10
Processed fruits and vegetables	
Candied fruit and vegetables	2000
Dried fruit (in fruit bars etc)	3000
Desiccated coconut	50
Ginger	750
Mixed dried fruit (in cakes)	3000
Imitation fruit (e.g. cherries)	3000
Apples and potatoes for manufacturing	200
Fruit and vegetable preparation for manufacturing	1000
Fruit and vegetable preparation incl pulp	350
Avocado, frozen	300
Dried vegetables	3000
Carrots, dried (in cake)	3000
Potatoes (hot chips, french fries)	200
Gelatine	
Gelatine (during manufacture)	750
Grain products and pasta	
Softening of corn kernels for starch	60
Meat	
Deli meats	500
Minced beef	illegal but it happens
Sausages and sausage meat (raw)	500
Edible casings	500
Sugars and syrups	
Glucose syrup	450
Molasses	450
Sweet sauces, toppings, syrups	
Fruit toppings, syrups	350

Sulphites in US foods

Alcoholic beverages	Wine, beer, cocktail mixes, wine coolers
Baked goods	Cookies, crackers, mixes with dried fruit or vegetables, pie crust, pizza crust, flour tortillas
Beverage bases	Dried citrus fruit beverage mixes
Condiments and relishes	Horseradish, onion and pickle relishes, pickles, olives, salad dressing mixes, wine vinegar
Confections and frostings	Brown, raw, powdered or white sugar derived from sugar beet
Dairy product analogues	Filled milk (skim milk enriched with vegetable oils)
Fish and shellfish	Canned clams; fresh, frozen, canned or dried shrimps; frozen lobster, scallops, dried cod
Fresh fruit and vegetables	Banned except for fresh pre-cut potatoes and sulphur dioxide used as a fungicide on grapes
Processed fruits	Canned, bottled or frozen fruit juices (including lemon, lime, grape, apple); dried fruit; canned, bottled or frozen dietetic fruit or fruit juices; maraschino cherries, glazed fruit
Processed vegetables	Vegetable juices; canned vegetables (including potatoes); pickled vegetables (including sauerkraut, cauliflower and peppers); dried vegetables; instant mashed potatoes; frozen potatoes; potato salad
Gelatins, puddings, fillings	Fruit fillings, flavoured and unflavoured gelatin, pectin, jelling agents
Grain products and pasta	Cornstarch, modified food starch, spinach pasta, gravies, hominy, breading, batters, noodle/rice mixes
Jams and jellies	Jams and jellies
Nuts and nut products	Shredded coconut
Plant protein products	Soy protein products
Snack foods	Dried fruits snacks, trail mixes, filled crackers
Soup and soup mixes	Canned soups, dried soup mixes
Sweet sauces, toppings, syrups	Corn syrup, maple syrup, fruit toppings, high-fructose corn syrup, pancake syrup, molasses
Tea	Instant tea, liquid tea concentrates

EATING OUT

For children, social occasions are likely to involve sausages—ask your school to provide preservative-free sausages (p. 248), or take your own. Avoid fries and hot chips. Fruit drinks and cordials are another major source of sulphites for young children. If you are going to eat at McDonald's, Rick recommends Chicken McNuggets (for people who don't react to antioxidants in oil). Drink milk or water. If you don't react to salicylates, he suggests pure orange juice and make your own dressing from honey and mustard.

It is easiest to eat at a few places that you know well. Ask about ingredients. Plain foods like steak or grilled fish and jacket potatoes are safest. Avoid commercial soups, dips, sauces, gravies and dressings. Liz suggests:

> It is really trial and error. I stick to things that are as fresh and as natural as possible. Chinese and Thai food is okay for me especially if they use lots of vegies and I always go where they don't use MSG. I avoid takeaway food as much as possible, as most pre-prepared foods have metabisulphite in them. If I must eat out, I choose salad on rolls or brown rye and avoid dressings. I don't eat takeaway pizzas, preferring to make my own so I have control over what goes into them. Before ordering anything when out, ask what has gone into it. If there are any doubts, don't order it. You soon get to know what you can and can't eat.

In the US, some of Rick's nosulfite but not failsafe recommendations are: *for breakfast*, waffles, pancakes or hotcakes with honey; *as an appetiser*, potato skins (no dressing); *in Italian restaurants*, avoid pizza and choose simple pasta with readily identifiable ingredients; at the Mexican *El Torita* chain, try corn tortillas, crisp tacos, refried beans, rice and tamales. For more details visit Rick's website: http://members. aol.com/nosulfites.

WHO'S WATCHING?

In Australia, sulphites are not permitted on fresh fish. One mother reported, 'We know if a food contains sulphites because my son has trouble breathing within a minute of eating it. Most fish is OK but occasionally he reacts.' Prawns—including those in seafood cocktails—always contain sulphites to preserve colour. The maximum permitted level is 30 ppm, but how well is it monitored? A seafood worker explained that they used 'metta' (sodium metabisulphite)—a white powder sprinkled over large quantities of fresh prawns by people wearing rubber gloves. Some prawns must have higher readings than others.

While we were testing recipes for my last book, my husband noticed that there were no sulphites listed on the brand of glucose syrup available in our supermarket. As a food technologist, he knows that glucose syrup contains sulphites. One of his first jobs was monitoring the levels of sulphites in glucose syrup. He commonly found levels up to four times over the legal limit. He contacted the company. They assured him they were using up old labels and would list it on the next labels. Two years on, however, nothing has changed.

WINE WITHOUT WHEEZE

Is it possible to make a decent sulphite-free wine? Wine buff Max Allen thinks so. He devoted an entire column in the *Australian Magazine* to a rave review of the 1999 Happs PF Red from Margaret River (www.happs.com.au). Preservative-free wine is not suitable for salicylate responders or even extra sensitive sulphite responders. Stick to your gin and tonic, whisky and soda, and vodka.

BE AWARE

Food regulators seem concerned with preventing deaths and severe reactions from sulphites, not asthma as such. They suggest:
- Never assume a food is safe to eat.
- If the food is packaged, read the label.
- If food is not packaged, e.g. sausages or deli meat, check ingredients with the manager.

- When eating out, check ingredients with the waiter or manager. Avoid foods listed on p. 188–89. If you want to eat potatoes when you're out, order a baked potato rather than fries, hash browns, mashed potatoes or any dish that involves peeling the potato first. For a snack, potato crisps are safe, fries are not.
- Always carry your blue puffer. If you have ever had a severe reaction to sulphites, carry injectable adrenaline with you.

But you shouldn't have to go through all this. As long ago as 1984, independent scientists from the Center for Science in the Public Interest recommended that sulphites be banned. In the meantime, technologists have developed more alternatives. In my opinion, sulphites, except in wines, should be banned now.

How to avoid MSG

Flavour enhancers (620–625)		Natural flavourings
620	L-glutamic acid	Flavours
621	Monosodium L-glutamate (MSG)	Kombu extract
622	Monopotassium L-glutamate	Yeast extract
623	Calcium di-L-glutamate	Accent
624	Monoammonium L-glutamate	Ajinomoto
625	Magnesium di-L-glutamate	Zest
HVP	Hydrolysed vegetable protein (up to 20% MSG)	Gourmet powder
HPP	Hydrolysed plant protein (up to 20% MSG)	Chinese seasoning

DON'T EXPECT TO FIND 'MSG' ON THE LABEL

In Australia, MSG is usually listed as flavour enhancer (621). It can also be added in other ways, such as yeast extract, or as part of an ingredient called Hydrolysed Plant Protein (HPP). This can be expressed in many combinations of words, for example, instead of *Plant* it can be *Vegetable*, or any kind of plant such as soy protein.

Since MSG is classified as a *flavour enhancer*, it is legal for the ingredients list on cheese snacks, for example, to boast *No Preservatives, No Artificial Colours, No Artificial Flavours* when the product can actually contain three doses of MSG (listed as *Flavour Enhancer 621, Hydrolysed Vegetable Protein* and *Yeast*

Extract) as well as two other flavour enhancers. The problem is that reactions are related to the size of the dose, and the dose from a concentrate can be much bigger than the dose you would eat in a food which contains naturally occurring glutamates.

LOOK FOR SOME FORM OF MSG IN FOODS SUCH AS THE FOLLOWING:

Flavoured chips and snacks • noodles and snacks with flavour packs or sachets • savoury biscuits e.g. with BBQ or pizza flavour • soups • soup stocks (stock cubes) • frozen dinners • sauces in a packet • gravies • Crumbing mixes • Seasoned salt • slimmers meals • backpacker freeze dried meals • deli meats • frozen turkey • frozen meat pies • fresh sausages (thin BBQ sausages from a major supermarket) • bottled sauces, (in one soy sauce, the major ingredient after water is HVP—naturally brewed soy sauce is the last ingredient, forming only 2.5% of the product).

SUPERMARKET FOODS LIKELY TO BE FREE OF MSG

Sweet biscuits
Sweets
Dairy products including icecream
Breakfast cereals
Rice, oats, flour, pasta
Dried beans and lentils
Fresh meat, fish and plain chicken
Eggs
Most fresh, frozen or canned fruit and vegetables right now (but see box following)

MSG IN FRUIT AND VEGIES

In the US, a spray containing nearly 30% L–glutamic acid (620) was recently approved as a 'plant growth and crop yield enhancer'. The product, called *AuxiGro WP Plant Metabolic Primer* has already been sprayed on lettuce, tomatoes, potatoes and peanuts. Other crops have been registered for use. For more details, see www.truthinlabeling.org.

FAST FOOD RESTAURANTS

Expect fast food to contain MSG, from meat toppings on pizza to batter on fried chicken (McDonald's provide a useful product ingredient list on their website www.mcdonalds.com). Barbecue chicken will have flavour enhancers in seasoning on the skin. Your best bet is unbattered, uncrumbed, grilled fish.

OTHER RESTAURANTS

Avoid Chinese restaurants which use MSG unless you are content to limit yourself to stir-fried vegetables on boiled rice. Some claim to avoid MSG. Can we believe them? At an Indonesian restaurant with a clear sign 'No MSG', I asked 'does this dish contain MSG?' The woman smiled. 'Only a little bit,' she said.

Thai restaurants don't always use MSG but they always have chili sauce. If the chili sauce comes out of a bottle, you need to read the label. Staff may be reluctant to admit that their food is not made on the premises, so ask straight out 'may I see the label on the bottle/packet?'

MSG is not limited to Asian restaurants. Avoid prepackaged foods and crumbing (e.g. prawn cutlets) or seasoning mixes (e.g. veal parmigiana). Be very suspicious of any soups, sauces, gravies or dressings. Even an old-fashioned Australian meal like roast chicken at the club is likely to have MSG in the gravy—check out the gravy premixes next time you are in the supermarket.

You need to ask about MSG, but general staff in large chains and cafeterias probably won't know. Even staff in smaller places genuinely may not know whether HVP or soy sauce and fish sauces are used for flavouring. A woman was surprised when her failsafe daughter had reacted two hours after a meal of plain roast turkey, boiled rice and plain lettuce in a café, despite assurances from the staff. When I checked the local supermarket, all except one brand of frozen turkey breasts contained some form of MSG.

The best way to eat out is to find a small restaurant which has friendly, helpful staff. Ask them whether food is prepared on the premises. Identify a few safe dishes, and stick to them. Some clubs frequented by seniors have been horrified when their clientele reported reactions and have agreed to switch to MSG-free gravy and sauces.

FOODS WHICH CONTAIN NATURAL MSG
Sensitive people may also react to glutamates which occur naturally in the following foods:
- Broccoli, champignon, green peas, mushroom, spinach, tomatoes and especially tomato products—tomato juice, tomato sauce, vegetable juice
- Plums, prunes, grapes and grape products—raisins, sultanas, wine
- Soy sauce, soy paste, miso, tempeh
- Brandy, liqueur, port, rum, sherry, wine
- Yeast extracts like Vegemite
- Meat extracts like Bonox
- Fish pastes like anchovy paste
- All tasty cheeses
- Sauces like soy, BBQ, worcestershire

How to avoid food colours
POTENTIALLY HARMFUL COLOURS
Avoid these colours during the elimination diet. Royal Prince Albert Hospital (RPAH) testing and many others have shown them to have potentially adverse effects.

Artificial colours (azo and/or coal tar dyes)
102	Tartrazine, yellow #5
104	Quinoline yellow, yellow #10
110	Sunset yellow, yellow #6
122	Azorubine, red #10, carmoisine
123	Amaranth, red #2
124	Ponceau 4R, red #4
127	Erythrosine, red #3
129	Allura, red #40
132	Indigotine, blue #2
133	Brilliant blue, blue #1
142	Food green, green #4

143   Fast green, green #3
151   Brilliant black
155   Brown HT

160b   Annatto extracts natural colour
Annatto is made from the seed coat of the tropical Annatto tree. 'Natural' is no guarantee of safety. More patients were affected by this colour than any artificial colours in a 1978 study.

PROCEED WITH CAUTION
120   Cochineal or carmines, red
This additive is unusual because it comes from the body of a South American insect. It is moderate in terms of food intolerance reactions, but severe life-threatening allergic reactions have been reported, especially, but not only, in dye workers. Avoid if you are atopic (susceptible to allergy).

150   Caramel
Caramel 150 may be divided into caramels 150a (plain or spirit caramel), 150b (caustic sulphite caramel), 150c (ammonia caramel) and 150d (ammonia sulphite caramel). Although caramel colour is considered safe by the RPAH, there are overseas reports of reactions to sulphite ammonia caramel in drinks by people who are very sensitive.

MODERATE—AVOID DURING THE ELIMINATION DIET
100   Turmeric or curcumin, yellow
140   Chlorophyll
141   Chlorophyll-copper
153   Carbon black, vegetable carbon (withdrawn in the US for
       possible cancer risk)
162   Beet red
163   Anthocyanins, red, blue, violet (from plants)
174   Silver
181   Tannic acid, brown

TOO NEW TO KNOW
Thirteen new colours were approved in the 2002 version of the Food Standards Code. The colours below are naturally derived, but that is no guarantee of safety.

103   Alkanet, pink
160c   Paprika deoresins and 160d lycopene, reds
160e   Beta-apo-carotenal and 160f apo-carotenic acid, yellows
161a   Flavoxanthin, 161b lutein, 161c kryptoxanthin
161d   Rubixanthin, 161e violoxanthin, 161f rhodoxanthin

FAILSAFE
101   Riboflavin (vitamin B2), yellow
160a   Beta-carotene, orange
170   Calcium carbonate, white
171   Titanium dioxide, white
172   Iron oxide—red, black, yellow

Read the ingredients list on every label. Look for colours in *obviously coloured foods* such as coloured breakfast cereals, confectionery, drinks, icecreams, yellow kebabs, yellow rice, red tandoori chicken, hot dogs and outrageously unnatural looking cheese and sauces.

Look for colours in *foods which are not obviously coloured*. Remember the breastfeeding mother in Chapter 4? She discovered she had been eating and feeding her toddler artificial colours in the following foods: potato, bread, yoghurt, canned soup, margarine, cough syrup, cakes, cake mixes, donuts, muffins, snack cakes, icecream, cookies, crackers, drink mixes, lemonade, pudding mix, boxed meals, rice and pasta dishes, cheesecake, butterscotch candy, jelly and chips. Do not assume that any food is uncoloured. Some white sweets, for example, appear to be white but contain a blue colour as well as salicylates. When you buy commercial garlic bread you are probably getting garlic margarine which contains artificial colour. Frozen french fries may contain colour.

There are also colours in *chocolate*, for example, two artificial reds and two artificial yellows in a brand of chocolate biscuits, six artificial colours in chocolate icypoles; look also in chocolate cake mixes, chocolate drink mixes and any other chocolate products.

Annatto natural colour appears in a very wide range of foods including yoghurt, icecream, breakfast cereals, biscuits and cheese, especially if labelled '*natural*', '*no artificial colours*', '*creamy*', '*lite*' or '*wholesome*', as well as hot dog skins, etc.

Don't forget colours in both prescription and over-the-counter *medications*, including throat lozenges and vitamins. Medications are not as well labelled as foods, which is really saying something. Vitamin manufacturers do not have to declare colours. Unless the label specifically says, 'no artificial colours, no annatto', you will have to phone and ask.

When eating out, assume that foods have harmful colours in them (for example, batter on fish) unless they are very plain (for example, steak), or you know it is safe. It's always safest to ask.

Remember also that colours can be absorbed through the skin and the eyes. Beware of coloured toiletries, coloured bubble bath and soaps, enemas, lotions and for children, coloured play-dough.

As with drugs, food additive testing is no guarantee of safety. Food additives have to cause cancer in rats before they will be withdrawn. New food colours are approved faster than allergy clinics can test them. I have divided colours into five categories. Remember that food colours are not necessary—they are only cosmetic. No-one will be affected if colours are omitted but many will be ill and some may even die when colours are used.

How to avoid benzoates

210   Benzoic acid
211   Sodium benzoate
212   Potassium benzoate
213   Calcium benzoate

Benzoate preservatives (210–213) occur naturally in many berries, fruits and vegetables—avoided in the failsafe diet—and sharp natural yoghurts. Like everything extracted from nature, as additives they are more concentrated and cause more problems.

Benzoates are commonly used as preservatives in drinks, from soft drinks and sports drinks, to fruit flavoured cordials, tomato juice and fruit juices, as well as fruit flavoured topping, low-joule jams, non-dairy dips and fish marinades. Read every label. Pure fruit juice, regular Coca-Cola, 7UP, some Schweppes lemonade, Schweppes tonic water and soda water are benzoate free.

When eating out, ask for your drinks by known brand, for example, Schweppes tonic if requesting a gin and tonic, other tonics are not preservative-free. Benzoates are also used in many medications which come as a syrup or solution. Tablets are safer.

How to avoid bread preservatives

280   Propionic acid
281   Sodium propionate
282   Calcium propionate (the most commonly used in breads)
283   Potassium propionate
—   whey powder which has been cultured with propionibacteria (you can't tell from the label, so avoid any bread with whey powder)

The bread preservative is one of the most difficult additives to avoid because its use is widespread in one of our most basic foods, our daily bread. In less than a generation, most Australians have gone from eating none of this additive to eating it every day.

Propionates (preservatives 280–283) occur naturally in small amounts in many foods and dairy products like Swiss cheese. In small amounts they are not harmful but, as with other additives, the effects are dose related and cumulative. Very few people will be affected by two slices of preserved bread but effects can build up slowly and unnoticeably.

Nearly all commercial bread now contains propionates, usually calcium propionate (282), including many specialty breads like pita bread and Indian breads. Ironically, this preservative does not keep your bread fresh. Calcium propionate (282) is added to inhibit the growth of mould. There is no mould on a freshly baked loaf of bread, so why use a mould inhibitor? If manufacturers are prepared to keep their work benches and slicer blades clean and mould-free, by wiping over with vinegar every day, there would be no problem. This is time-consuming and modern bakers would rather 'fog' their bakeries with a less effective chemical spray. Putting hot loaves in plastic bags makes the problem worse. Preservative 282 is for the convenience of the manufacturer not the consumer.

Read the ingredients on every label. When you buy bread in a sandwich shop, bakery or restaurant, assume it contains 282 and ask to see the bread label or in a bakery, the bag of premix. If mould inhibitors or preservatives 280–282 are listed, *refuse to buy*. You can ask for the sandwich filling to be served in a takeaway container. Brumbys (www.brumbys.com.au) and Bakers Delight (www.bakersdelight.com.au) are Australia-wide hot bread chains selling preservative-free bread, see phone directories or websites for an outlet near you. In Tasmania, see Banjos (www.banjos.com.au). Otherwise, look at the specialty breads in your supermarket. Sometimes you can find one without preservatives. Note that calcium propionate can be cultured naturally in whey powder as a method of using preservatives without labelling, so avoid breads with whey powder. Breads with vinegar may affect sensitive people as badly as propionates. You can buy a breadmaker and make your own bread the traditional way, from flour, water, yeast, sugar, oil and salt, or use Laucke's breadmaker premixes, available in most supermarkets, see www.laucke.com.au. See my website www. fedupwithfoodadditives.info for more suggestions.

Reactions to propionates are probably the most difficult to identify of any additive reaction because they build up so slowly. In Australia, I have not yet received complaints about reactions to propionates in other products such as cheese or fruit juice, but a mother in the US who was keeping her son on a propionate-free diet noticed a big reaction after a pizza. When she asked, staff told her their pizza crusts were propionate-free but the cheese was 'just loaded with it'.

In New Zealand, most bread is still 282-free, although most contain antioxidants BHA or TBHQ. In the US, we didn't ever find any sliced white loaves without calcium propionate. We bought specialty bread like Italian or French.

How to avoid nitrates, nitrites

249   Potassium nitrite
250   Sodium nitrite
251   Sodium nitrate
252   Potassium nitrate

Nitrates and nitrites are used as curing agents, colour fixatives and preservatives in meat. They are easy to avoid. Eat fresh meats and avoid processed or cured meats like ham, bacon, devon, pressed chicken and other luncheon meats, frankfurters, saveloys, hot dogs, canned cured meat like tinned ham and corned beef.

Current regulations make you wonder about food industry. According to *Additive Code Breaker*, for the purpose of food regulations nitrates and nitrites are not classed as preservatives. However, foods containing these additives may not be described as preservative-free.

How to avoid antioxidants

These additives won a Worst Additive competition on my website because they are in nearly all processed foods and many are unlabelled under the 5 per cent labelling loophole. The words 'contains no preservatives' won't protect you because technically these additives are not preservatives. The person who submitted the winning entry wrote:

> Antioxidants are secret unless you go to extreme lengths to ask the supplier of the food and then the manufacturer of the contents . . . what hope have we got if such nasty additives are *hidden* in our foods?

ANTIOXIDANTS

310   Propyl gallate
311   Octyl gallate
312   Dodecyl gallate
319   tert-Butylhydroquinone, tBHQ
320   Butylated hydroxyanisole, BHA
321   Butylated hydroxytoluene, BHT

SAFE ALTERNATIVES

300	Ascorbic acid (Vitamin C)
301	Sodium ascorbate
302	Calcium ascorbate
303	Potassium ascorbate
304	Ascorbyl palmitate
306	Mixed tocopherols (Vitamin E)
307	dl-a-Tocopherol
308	g-Tocopherol
309	d-Tocopherol
—	opaque containers

Look for these additives in cooking oils, margarines, lards and any other fats or oils. Then look for the products which contain these and you will start to understand the problem. Nearly every processed food contains some kind of fat or oil. It doesn't matter whether the ingredient label says vegetable oil, a specific oil like canola or sunflower, fats of vegetable origin, or beef tallow— unless they list some of the safe alternatives, they will probably contain one of these harmful additives. Small amounts don't affect people unless they are very sensitive, but if you eat them every day, effects will build up.

THE 5 PER CENT LABELLING LOOPHOLE

If the amount of an ingredient in a food is less than 5 per cent of the food (such as 4.5 per cent sunflower oil added to soymilk), a food additive (such as antioxidant TBHQ, 319) in that ingredient does not have to be included in the ingredients list on the label unless the food additive is performing a technological function in the final food. Who decides if the additive is performing a tech-nological function? The food manufacturers. What if consumption of the unlisted food additive can affect consumers? Too bad.

Unlike commercial oils, at least most cooking oils for home use in Australia are antioxidant-free. Read the ingredient label. New Zealanders are even worse off. Consumers are told their fats and oils have to be 'protected' by these potentially harmful additives. It is very difficult to buy pure cooking oil in New Zealand supermarkets.

When you eat out, any oils used to cook your food will almost certainly contain at least one of these potentially harmful additives, so avoid fried foods. Sulphites are not the only problem in french fries.

Check the ingredients of your pantry. Look at your margarine, dairy blend, crackers, biscuits, bread, baked goods, croissants, potato crisps, snack foods, muesli bars, crushed garlic in oil, soymilk and other processed foods. Any food which contains vegetable oils may contain these antioxidants and they are not necessarily labelled. Eat these products every day and you will never know what has affected you.

I discovered this when I carried out research, published in a medical journal, using the failsafe diet for behaviour. In the first stage, two of the children failed to improve on the diet. I noticed that both were eating large quantities of a particular biscuit. A call to the manufacturer revealed that the biscuits contained vegetable oil with unlabelled BHA. As soon as we removed these items from the diet, the children improved.

Failsafers were outraged when a health food company started to use a sunflower oil containing TBHQ in their soymilks without any mention on the label. Many families using this soymilk gradually realised that the failsafe diet had stopped working for them. When the mother who discovered this change switched her son to another soymilk, he started doing much better. She said, 'I'm so angry about manufacturers getting away with what they put in their foods.'

Customer relations consultants at the company acknowledged that TBHQ can cause problems in some sensitive people, yet our food regulations keep its presence in our foods undisclosed. When the company eventually switched to an oil with failsafe antioxidants, they faced another problem. How could they let food intolerant customers know that their soymilk was again safe to drink? Since TBHQ had never been declared, there was no way of telling it was gone again from the ingredient list on the label.

To avoid harmful antioxidants, you must stick to the products listed on the shopping list and read the product updates on

www.fedupwithfoodadditives.info. If you want to eat any
unlisted products containing any fats or oils, phone the manufacturers and ask specifically about each of the gallates, TBHQ
and BHA listed previously on p. 202–03. We shouldn't have to
rely on word of mouth to judge the safety of food products.
Public health is not protected when parents have to go to these
lengths to safeguard their children.

BHT
For many years, BHT (321) has been added to cling film plastic
food wrap and to package liners of ready-to-eat cereals because
it migrates into foods and helps to prevent rancidity. In the US,
BHT is permitted in both cereals and cereal packages at a level
of 50 mg/kg compared to 2 mg/kg in Australian packaging.
Regulations are currently changing and it is hard to say how
much BHT will be permitted in the future. The highest dose of
BHT in Australian food is 200 mg/kg in chewing gum.

How to avoid salicylates
Salicylates are natural pesticides produced by plants to protect
themselves from insects and diseases, so any food, colour,
flavour, perfume or drug derived from plants might contain
salicylates. This includes fruit, vegetables, nuts, herbs, spices,
tea, coffee, beer, wine, juice, fruit, licorice and mint flavours,
honey, eucalyptus and aspirin. Salicylate levels decrease with
ripening. Despite the food industry's best efforts, and lucky for
us, there are still some foods low in salicylates (see p. 219–31).
   People who are exceptionally sensitive to salicylates may not
be able to manage the full list of failsafe foods and will have to
be careful of exposure to inhaled salicylates in perfumes and
other scents (see p. 218).

How to avoid amines
As an amine responder myself, I have found amines more difficult to understand than any other food chemical. Amines are
produced by the breakdown of proteins or by fermentation,
which means that they change depending on food freshness,

handling, and the passing of time. While fresh meat sits in your refrigerator, amines are increasing. Fish more than one day old, or fish which has been frozen more than a few weeks, can be very high in amines. Long cooking or charring on a barbecue can increase amines. Foods affected by fermentation include not only alcoholic beverages but also sharp natural yoghurts, sauer-kraut and sourdough or long-rise yeast-free breads.

There are large amounts of amines in cheese, chocolate, wine, processed fish, beer and yeast extracts like Vegemite. Some fruit and vegetables also contain amines: see the full list (p. 219–31) and hints regarding extra sensitivity to amines (p. 277).

How to avoid added flavours

Artificial flavours and 'natural flavours' are both man-made additives. The only difference is that natural flavours must be derived entirely from natural products. Natural and artificial flavours can end up containing exactly the same chemicals. You can't tell what's in them because flavour formulas are top secret.

A typical artificial strawberry flavour—found in milkshakes and children's medicines—will contain about 50 chemicals, including methyl salicylate and a form of benzoate. It's actually not so different from what you might find in a natural straw-berry, but because man-made flavours are cheap, it is easy to add a lot more than you would ever eat in a serve of a natural food. Maybe that's why some children react so badly to added flavours in foods and medicines such as antibiotic syrup.

How do you avoid added flavours? Avoid any processed food with added flavours except those listed in the shopping list. Or eat in very limited amounts. Remember that the effects of food chemicals are usually not obvious. They creep up on you.

How to avoid cow's milk

Reactions to dairy foods can be either food intolerance or true allergy. During your elimination diet you need to avoid all sources of dairy foods—milk, butter, margarine with dairy products, ghee, cheese, cream, sour cream, yoghurt, buttermilk, skimmed milk, low-fat milk, milk powder, whey, condensed milk, evaporated milk, malted milk, custard, icecream and commercial products containing these or any mention of milk or dairy on the label, until you have confirmed the problem and discovered the extent of the sensitivity.

People with intolerance can generally get away with a certain amount of dairy products, but be careful. One failsafe mother, who knew her three-year-old's respiratory problems and asthma were associated with dairy foods, allowed lots of dairy treats during a long school holiday. In the last week, her son caught a virus, became wheezy and was hospitalised with pneumonia. This was followed by recurring ear infections requiring antibiotics and a reaction to the benzoate preservative in the antibiotic syrup—a typical chain of events provoked by dairy products in this child.

ALTERNATIVES
These include soymilk, dairy free margarine (Nuttelex), soy yoghurt, soy cream cheese and soy icecream: see failsafe substitutes, p. 235 and nutrition, p. 75. People with milk allergy can be allergic to soy as well. If soy is also a problem, calcium fortified rice milk is an option. For babies, there are special formulas (Pepti Junior, Alfare and Neocate). Your dietitian can advise you about nutrition.

TRUE ALLERGY
Children with a true allergy to cow's milk can be very sensitive indeed. For more details, see www.allergyfacts.com.

How to avoid eggs
Although eggs are failsafe from the food intolerance point of view, egg is the most common food allergy in babies and young children. It is also the most likely to be grown out of after the age of three. In high risk babies, avoidance of egg in the mother's diet through late pregnancy and breastfeeding, and in the baby's diet for the first year, may avoid sensitisation.

Egg white is more likely to cause problems than yolk but

both can be implicated. Life-threatening reactions to egg are rare but can occur. Babies with egg allergy usually react with eczema, but they are at increased risk of developing asthma later on. People with egg allergy often have an aversion to all egg-containing foods such as cakes and custards except icecream. For a list of egg-containing ingredients and foods, see www.allergyfacts.com.au.

SOME FAILSAFE EGG SUBSTITUTES
These will work best in moist recipes like muffins. Replace one egg with:
- 1 or 2 tsp commercial egg replacer (*Egglike* or *No Egg*)
- 1 tsp bakers yeast dissolved in ¼ cup warm water
- 1 tbspn pear jam or pear puree
- 1½ tbsp water plus 1½ tbsp failsafe oil plus 1 tsp baking powder.

How to avoid peanuts
For people with food intolerance, peanuts contain salicylates and amines and are therefore not permitted on the failsafe diet. For people with allergies, peanut allergy is the most dangerous because exposure is hard to avoid, and even trace amounts can trigger life-threatening symptoms. The prevalence of peanut allergy is increasing.

AVOIDING PEANUT ALLERGY
Babies are most likely to become sensitised to peanuts through a mother who eats peanuts or peanut butter during late pregnancy and breastfeeding, through close contact (for example, kissing) with others who eat peanuts or peanut butter, or skin lotions containing peanut oils. Peanut butter is a particular problem because it is so sticky and residues can be spread. If your child is at high risk, you can choose to avoid peanuts and peanut butter in the last six weeks of pregnancy and during breastfeeding, have a peanut-free home and send your child to a peanut-free child-care centre—these are becoming more common. Delay the introduction of any peanut-containing foods or health care products

until after baby's first birthday. The allergy usually becomes obvious the first time the child eats peanut butter.

People who are allergic to peanuts may be allergic to other nuts or sesame seeds or, rarely, to other legumes like lentils, beans and peas. More commonly, other nuts, as well as chocolate and chocolate products, are contaminated with peanuts and should be avoided. For a list of peanut-containing ingredients and foods, see www.allergyfacts.com.au.

How to avoid seafood

For people with food intolerance, fresh white fish fillets are failsafe, and so are fresh oysters, squid and scallops (shellfish, not potato scallops). How can you be sure they are sulphite-free? You can't. The 1994 Market Basket Survey found some oysters contained sulphites. For people with a true allergy, see a list of fish-containing foods and sauces at www.allergyfacts.com.

How to avoid wheat and gluten

The link between asthma, wheat and/or gluten is mentioned in medical journals only with regard to exercise-induced anaphylaxis, but some failsafers report wheat or gluten-associated asthma.

> I did the whole failsafe diet very carefully, for months. It helped with other things, but my asthma didn't clear up until I avoided gluten as well. I've been asthmatic all my life, and needed steroids frequently until I went gluten-free. Now I've had several years without any medication.

ALLERGY OR INTOLERANCE?

True wheat allergies are not common and rarely life-threatening. Food intolerance reactions to wheat usually occur only in people with a family history of irritable bowel. As well as irritable bowel, symptoms can include upper airway congestion, rash, sleep disturbance and irritable behaviour.

People who need to avoid wheat can eat wheat-free rye bread, oats and barley as well as any gluten-free products.

Intolerance to gluten can be a sign of an autoimmune condition called coeliac disease (diagnosed by blood test and bowel biopsy), or gluten intolerance induced by overuse of antibiotics or a gastrointestinal infection (confirmed by elimination and challenge). People who need to avoid gluten must avoid any products containing wheat, wheaten cornflour, rye, oats and barley, from bread and other baked goods to pastry, pasta, crumbed or battered foods, sauces and thickeners.

ALTERNATIVES

Rice, corn, potatoes, buckwheat, arrowroot, tapioca, sago, millet, amaranth and quinoa are all gluten-free substitutes for wheat. Chefs in restaurants and cafes often have a good understanding of gluten intolerance, and there are an increasing number of gluten-free products available in supermarkets. Gluten-free flours may contain sulphites, sometimes unlabelled. For more information and gluten-free recipes, see the *Failsafe Cookbook*.

20 Managing other asthma triggers

House dust, pollens, animals and exercise are some of the top triggers reported by adult asthmatics. Others include viral infections like colds and flu, dramatic weather changes, irritants and strong smells like cigarette smoke, perfumes and chemicals, excessive laughing or crying, emotional stress, thunderstorms, air conditioning, mould, hay, newly cut grass, windy days, alcohol and some foods. For children, viruses and—unexpectedly—laughter are considered to be common triggers.

As explained elsewhere in this book, continual exposure to food chemicals like sulphites can create irritable airways. Environmental triggers like house dust can then tip you over the edge into an obvious reaction. Many asthmatics report that they no longer react to former triggers after going failsafe.

Skin prick testing will typically screen for allergens like house dust mite, common grass pollens, cats and dogs and moulds. Allergies are most likely to develop through constant exposure in susceptible people. Asthmatics are advised that the best way to deal with asthma triggers is to avoid them, but this is not what you want to do with laughter and exercise.

Laughter

A study at Sydney Children's Hospital suggests that laughter is a major asthma trigger in children. Over a six-month period, almost one third of children who were taken to the emergency department because they were suffering from an asthma attack had laughter-triggered asthma. Laughter while watching a movie caused the biggest reduction in peak flow.

What do kids do while watching a movie? They also consume additive-laden junk food, although the researchers didn't consider that. I checked the food at a typical cinema. Despite a lack of labels, 99 per cent of the sweets obviously contained artificial colours, icecreams are highly likely to contain additives, all soft drinks contain additives or salicylates, and see the comment regarding popcorn in the box below. Here are some alternatives:

Foods to watch movies with—take your own: failsafe chips and sweets (p. 237).

Foods to buy there: bottle of spring water; Crunchie Bars, Violet Crumble Bars, Maltesers (these are not failsafe but they are better than anything else).

FAQ: Is popcorn failsafe?
A. Home–cooked popcorn is not failsafe because corn is high in salicylates. Commercial popcorn has the extra problem of additives. At one cinema, an attendant explained how they add a premix powder. 'I wouldn't eat it,' she said. 'There's a lot of powder, I don't know what's in it.' From supermarket labels, I would guess artificial yellow colour, artificial flavour, and anti-oxidants (TBHQ 319 or BHA 320) in the vegetable oil.

Viruses, colds and flu

Viruses, especially colds and flu, are often reported as an asthma trigger. Frequent colds and flu are a symptom of food intolerance. The longer you stay failsafe, the more you will notice how well your family is, and how infrequently you all catch colds. The improvement will occur gradually over many months. Eventually, you will notice that the members of your family rarely catch colds and flu and when they do, asthma does not result.

IF YOU DO GET A COLD

- **Avoid unnecessary medications**, especially those containing artificial colours, flavours and preservatives, that is, *most* cold remedies. The Oxfam village health care handbook suggests, 'People will get well from most sicknesses—including the common cold and flu—by themselves, without need for medicines'. We in the affluent West could learn a lot from it.

- For a fever, **rest and drink lots of fluids**. The latest medical thinking is that fever is the body's way of healing itself and the fever should be allowed to run its course. Always consult a doctor when necessary.

- For mucus, **drink lots of fluids**. This will loosen mucus and get it moving out of your body. Water is the best drink. You can also try home-made chicken soup and hot 'lemon' drink (p. 246).

- **Eat well**. If you want to give your child treats, make them failsafe treats, especially fruit and vegetables (from the moderate column if you react to salicylates).

- **Breathe hot water vapours** to loosen mucus. Put your head over a basin of very hot water. Place a large towel or sheet over your head to catch the vapours as they rise. Breathe the vapours deeply for 15 minutes several times a day. Some people like to add menthol preparations but these are high in salicylates and definitely not failsafe. Hot water alone works just as well. A hot bath also helps.

- **Gargle with warm salt water** for sore throat.

- For a stuffed-up nose, **use salt water**. Pharmacies sell ready-made saline called Narium Nasal Mist to spray into nostrils as required, or you can make your own by mixing 2 tsp of salt and 1 tsp bicarbonate of soda in one litre of boiled water and allow to cool. Transfer to a spray container or apply to the nostrils with a dropper.

- **To soothe a ticklish throat**, suck slowly on a hard sweet like additive-free caramel or butterscotch like Werthers Original Butter Candy.

- **When medications are essential** for relief of pain and fever, white paracetamol (Panadol, Tylenol) tablets are failsafe and Bisolvon white tablets—not elixir—are helpful mucolytics (they breakdown thickened mucus). The dose for children aged 1–3 is half a tablet 3 times daily.

- **If antibiotics are necessary**, avoid the artificial colours, flavours and preservatives that go with them, p. 84.

Dust mites

House dust is a major allergy trigger. When asthmatics notice dusting, vacuuming or bedmaking as their triggers they are usually—but not always—reacting to dust-mites and their droppings. Dust mites thrive in humidity. They live in soft furnishings like carpets, cushions, quilts and mattresses, stored clothes and soft toys.

The family of a four-year-old girl chose to do the elimination diet because their daughter's nose was so stuffed up she couldn't talk properly. On the diet, she improved so much that they could then identify environmental triggers like perfumed soap and shampoo. But she was still stuffed up first thing in the morning. When the soft toys hanging over her bed were removed, she woke up the next morning 'as clear as a bell'.

What can you do to reduce house dust mites?

Reduce humidity with good ventilation—wide open windows except during pollen season—or constant airconditioning. Clothes dryers, drying washing, humidifiers, and fish tanks will all increase humidity. Dust mites can dehydrate and come back to life when the humidity increases.

Reduce dust mite habitats with hard floors and washable rugs instead of carpets. Use washable cotton covers for beds instead of doonas.

Trap dust mites inside commercially available mattress covers and pillow covers. Every bed a child uses—including the parents' bed—will need to be covered.

Kill dust mites in water hotter than 55°C (too hot to put your hand in) or clothes dryers. Put soft toys in a plastic bag in the freezer overnight. This will kill the dust mites. Wash in cold water to remove allergens including dead mites and their droppings. Wash all bedding including mattress covers every four to six weeks.

Take your medication with you when visiting friends and relatives whose houses may have more dust mites than yours.

'We were visiting friends and there was a group of us all sleeping on the living room floor. I spent all night sitting up because I was having trouble breathing. I didn't realise it at the time, but I know now that was the first time I had asthma due to dust mites.'

Pollen

Pollen is a major trigger factor for allergies. A Melbourne study suggests that hayfever sufferers and asthmatics may be affected by different particle sizes. Big pollen particles are likely to lodge in the nose and eyes causing hayfever symptoms while smaller particles are likely to penetrate the airways, producing asthma.

The biggest risk for asthmatics is a combination of pollen plus water. Wet pollen grains burst, releasing thousands of tiny starch granules. During the pollen season, days following rain are especially dangerous for asthmatics. The average sunny day particle count of 1,000 per cubic metre of air can jump to 54,000 on a day after rain.

WHAT YOU CAN DO

Tighten up on your diet during the pollen season. Other than that, avoidance is the key. Stay indoors on windy days and during and after rain in the pollen season. On sunny days, the best time to go outside during pollen season is late afternoon— pollen counts peak in the morning after sunrise when the temperature rises. Don't hang wet washing outside on windy days or at night—it will end up covered in pollen. Don't smell the flowers—reactions can be delayed. Keep lawns short to prevent flowering.

FROM THE MEDICAL JOURNALS

'It is often possible to manage pollen allergies satisfactorily by giving attention to diet during the pollen season.'

Bass DJ, Clinically important pollens of NSW and the ACT, *Med J Aust*, 1984, 141(5):S13–14.

A LOW-POLLEN ENVIRONMENT

Californian horticulturalist Tom Ogren believes that pollen counts are increasing in cities all over the world because landscapers are choosing male plants that produce huge amounts of pollen to spread in the wind. Traditional insect-pollinated plants and female plants produce a lot less pollen in the air, but urban landscapers avoid female plants because their seeds and fruit make a mess when they fall.

Ogren recommends choosing plants for their allergy potential. The closer you are to the source of pollen, the more you're exposed. Plant low-allergy trees near windows, doors and decks. Some Australian natives, including Casuarinas and paperbarks, have high allergy rankings. More information at www.allergyfree-gardening.com.

Moulds and fungal spores

Exposure to moulds is usually highest outdoors. Lawn mowing, leaf raking, mouldy hay and compost can increase exposure to fungi. Indoors, exposure to moulds is highest in winter. Build up of moulds can be prevented by good ventilation, dry air and cleaning with anti-mould agents.

Animals

Asthmatics can be allergic to many kinds of animals from horses, cats and dogs to small furry animals like guinea pigs, rats and mice. An allergy to horses is an indication of a very sensitive person. It is much more serious than a reaction only to pollen.

The biggest problem with cats is allergenic particles in cat saliva—which can be widespread, not just on cats. Male cats are more allergenic than female cats and some cats are worse than others. Giving away your cat will not necessarily help. Cat allergens can last for six months or even years in the former home of a cat and can also be strong enough on a cat lover to affect a sensitive child.

Exercise

Exercise-induced asthma affects about 80 per cent of asthmatics but exercise is an asthma trigger you should not avoid. The beneficial effects of exercise are only now becoming fully understood. Exercise strengthens the immune system and protects against ageing.

Any exercise will do. Walking is as useful an exercise as jogging or running if you cover the same distance. It just takes longer. Since it is a form of breath training, swimming is thought to be particularly beneficial for asthmatics, although chemicals called chloramines in the air at indoor swimming pools have been linked with occupational asthma. Chloramines are formed by the interaction of pool chlorine and sweat and urine from swimmers' bodies.

There is much greater recognition of the role of foods in exercise-induced anaphylaxis than for exercise-induced asthma, but they are similar conditions. If you start your elimination diet now, by the time you get yourself organised into regular exercise, your failsafe diet should have kicked in, and exercise-induced asthma will no longer be a problem.

Latex

Latex allergy is a relatively newly recognised condition. See more details p. 142. Asthma is a possible reaction. People most at risk of developing an allergy to latex are those with asthma, eczema or hayfever. People with regular contact with latex are more likely to become sensitised. Reactions can be mild, such as rashes on hands, itchy swollen eyes and sneezing, but latex allergy can get worse with continued exposure. A life-threatening reaction may be the first sign of a latex allergy, particularly in children.

WHAT YOU CAN DO

Avoid latex in rubber gloves, surgical gloves (tell your doctor, dentist and hairdresser you have a latex allergy), new powdered latex swimming caps, balloons, pacifiers for babies, dental dams, catheters, face masks (including latex masks on spacers for asthmatics), condoms and contraceptive diaphragms, rubber tubing, rubber bands, elastic in clothes, rubber handles on racquets, rubber bathmats, natural rubber pillows and mattresses and bicycle tyres. For health care workers, all staff in the area will need to wear non-powdered gloves.

Perfumes and other chemicals

Exposure to toxic chemicals can trigger respiratory problems
and asthma in susceptible people. Some chemicals act as sensitisers, that is, exposure can make you more sensitive to other
chemicals. You can't avoid all chemicals, but you can reduce
your total load.

Choose low-scent deodorants, hair products, cosmetics and
washing powders, see alternatives (p. 239). Reduce your use of
strong-smelling household cleaners. You can do most cleaning
with vinegar, dishwashing liquid, dishwashing detergent and soda
bicarbonate. Avoid smells from new cars, carpets and soft furnishings like mattresses. Leave such items well ventilated in the
sun until the smell wears off. Reduce your use of pesticides on
your pet, for pests such as cockroaches, and on your garden. Especially avoid organophosphates like chlorpyrifos and diazinon. For
more details, see www.fedupwithfoodadditives.info.

21 Foods to eat, foods to avoid

Vegetables

EAT	AVOID S = salicylates A = amines G = glutamates		
LOW	MODERATE	HIGH	VERY HIGH
beans, green	asparagus S	alfalfa S	broadbean SA
brussels	beetroot S	artichoke S	cauliflower SA
sprouts	carrots S	capsicum S	eggplant SA
cabbage	Chinese	chili S	gherkin SA
(green, red)	greens S	chicory S	olive SA
celery	lettuce (except	corn S	
chives	iceberg) S	cucumber S	broccoli SAG
choko	marrow S	endive S	champignon
dried beans	parsnip S	onion S	SAG
dried peas	potato	radish S	mushroom SAG
garlic	(new, red) S	water	spinach SAG
leeks	pumpkin S	chestnut	rocket SAG
lentils	snow peas	(yambean) S	tomato SAG
lettuce, iceberg	(and sprouts) S	watercress S	
potato (large,	sweet potato S	zucchini S	
white, peeled)	turnip S		
shallots			
shoots,	green peas G		
bamboo			
sprouts, mung			
swedes			

Eat from the low column during your elimination diet. Since most food chemicals are in the skin or just underneath, peel vegetables thickly. Throw away the outer leaves of lettuce. Note that all dried beans—kidney, butter, borlotti, navy, garbanzo, etc—are failsafe except broadbeans. Potatoes should be large, white or dirty, brown. *Avoid* vegetables in the moderate, high and very high columns, especially tomatoes and tomato products, vegetable juices, vegetable stocks and pastes, canned soups, canned baked beans in sauce, pickled vegetables (SAG); flavoured bean mix (S); sulphites in dried packet soups, dehydrated peas, instant mashed potato; hot chips (fries) and potato gems (also antioxidant in oils), baby food in cans and jars.

Fruit

EAT	AVOID S = salicylates A = amines G = glutamates		
LOW	MODERATE	HIGH	VERY HIGH
pears, peeled, ripe, juicy, soft canned in syrup, or baby puree	apples (golden or red delicious) **S**	apples except delicious **S**	citrus except lemons (oranges, mandarins, grapefruit, pomelo, tangelo) **SA**
	custard apple **S**	berries except raspberries **S**	
	loquat **S**	currants (black, red) **S**	
	mango **S**		
	pears (unripe, unpeeled, canned in natural juice, nashi) **S**	melons (watermelon, rockmelon, honeydew) **S**	avocadoes **SA**
			dates **SA**
	persimmon **S**	stone fruit (apricot, cherry, nectarine, peach) **S**	kiwi fruit **SA**
	rhubarb **S**		passionfruit **SA**
			pineapple **SA**
	banana **A**		raspberries **SA**
	pawpaw, yellow **A**	guava **S**	grapes **SAG**
	pawpaw, red **SA**	lychee **S**	plums **SAG**
		pomegranate **S**	prunes **SAG**
		rambutan **S**	raisins **SAG**
			sultanas **SAG**
		figs **SA**	
		lemons **SA**	
		sugar banana **SA**	

Eat from the low column. For salicylates, ripe is better. For amines, ripe is worse. Cooking does *not* reduce salicylates. *Avoid* fruits in the moderate, high and very high columns; any other fruits, fruit juice, cordials, dried fruits, fruit flavourings and toppings even when all natural; salty plums (SAG, colours and sulphites). Berries high in salicylates include blackberries, blue berries, boysenberries, cranberries, loganberries, mulberries and strawberries. Note that raspberries are rated *very high* in both salicylates and amines. Note that lemons are the only citrus rated *high* in salicylates and amines. Sugar bananas are the short, fat bananas also known as ladyfingers. Don't panic, the recipes will show you how to live without fruit, see Chapter 22.

Cereals, grains, flours

EAT	AVOID S = salicylates A = amines G = glutamates
LOW	HIGH
amaranth	Avoid all corn products except cornflour. Avoid
arrowroot	cornflakes, cornflake crumbs, popcorn, corn chips,
barley	tacos, cornmeal, wholegrain cornflour or maize
buckwheat	flour, polenta, cereals with corn (e.g. Nutrigrain) **S**
cornflour,	
refined	
cous cous	
malt	breakfast cereals with fruit, nuts, coconut (**SA**),
millet	honey (**S**), cocoa (**A**)
potato flour	
quinoa	
rice	basmati, jasmine, wild rice, flavoured rice **S**
rolled oats	commercial baby rice cereals **SA**
rye	
sago	canned spaghetti, coloured or flavoured noodles,
semolina	pasta **SAG**
soy flour	
spelt	breads with corn, dried fruit, seeds except poppy,
tapioca	breads with preservatives, mould inhibitors, flour
wheat	treatment agent 223, whey, vinegar preservatives
	202, 280–283 in bread, pita bread, rolls, muffins,
	crumpets, pizza base, breadcrumbs **SA**

Plain rice cereals, rice cakes and noodles, plain rolled oats, plain wheat cereals, plain uncoloured pasta and noodles, plain and poppyseed preservative-free bread and rolls, plain water crackers, crispbreads, crackers, plain biscuits, plain shortbread are OK, see shopping list. *Avoid* any bakery product containing unsuitable additives or ingredients such as fruit, spices especially cinnamon, chocolate, honey, corn, seeds except poppyseeds, or unsuitable oil, e.g. Christmas cakes and carrot cakes. Potato flour is preserved with sulphites. Maize cornflour may contain residues. Most disappears in the cooking process. Some people may need to avoid it. Food sensitive children and adults may do better on white bread than wholemeal bread.

Meat and seafood

EAT	AVOID S = salicylates A = amines G = glutamates	
LOW	HIGH	VERY HIGH
beef	aged beef **A**	anchovies **A**
veal	bacon, ham **A**	fish roe, caviar **A**
lamb	chicken skin, liver **A**	offal (liver, kidneys) **A**
rabbit	frozen fish **A**	pate (from liver) **A**
failsafe	meat juice in gravy,	*processed fish*
sausages	stews, stocks **A**	dried, pickled,
(p. 248)	pork **A**	salted, canned **A**
chicken (no		
skin)		*smoked products*
	non–white seafood	(meat, fish, chicken) **A**
fresh white fish	prawns **A**	
fresh crab	salmon **A**	self–basting turkey **G**
fresh lobster	sardines **A**	fish sauces,
fresh oysters	tuna **A**	marinades **SAG**
fresh mussels		fish pastes **SAG**
calamari		gravy **SAG**
sea scallops		*spiced meats*
		(devon, pressed
		chicken, meat pies,
		sausage rolls, salami,
		sausages, marinated
		meats, seasoned
		chicken) **SAG**

Eat from the low column during your elimination diet. Amines increase with age. Buy meat fresh and cook that day or use from the freezer within one month. Buy fish within 12 hours of catch and cook that day or freeze and use within 2 weeks. Freeze leftovers (e.g. roasts). Cooking increases amines (browning, grilling, charring, long slow cooking). Microwaving or pressure cooking is safer. *Avoid* processed meats and fish (nitrates in meats; amines in fish; salicylates and MSG in seasonings; amines, colours in fish fingers, crab sticks).

Dairy foods

EAT	AVOID S = salicylates A = amines G = glutamates	
LOW **dairy products, cow or goat**	HIGH	VERY HIGH
butter, salted, unsalted, ghee	dairy blend with unlisted antioxidants 319, 320	flavoured butters **S**
cream, fresh, sour, reduced, thickened		artificial creams
milk, plain, unflavoured, fresh, full–cream, low fat, skim, buttermilk, UHT, condensed, powdered, evaporated		flavoured milk, colours **S**
yoghurt, vanilla or natural, no annatto or artificial colour		yoghurts, icecream with colours, flavours **S**
icecream, vanilla, no colour		
fresh cheeses (white–cream, ricotta, farm, mascarpone, cottage, no preservatives, no flavours)	mild cheeses mozarella edam **A**	tasty cheeses brie, camembert, cheddar, parmesan, processed, swiss, vintage, fetta **AG**

If dairy is permitted, *avoid* artificial colours and annatto 160b in flavoured milks, yoghurt, icecream, custard and custard powder. Avoid fruit flavours (**S**). Vanilla is limited to 2 drops per day, approach vanilla flavoured yoghurts, soymilk and especially soy icecreams with caution. Some commercial custards and dairy desserts like creme caramel may be failsafe if colour and preservative-free. Extra sensitive amine responders will not manage sour cream or sharp natural yoghurt. Avoid cheese sticks (preservatives) and all yellow or aged cheeses.

Egg, non-dairy

EAT	AVOID S = salicylates A = amines G = glutamates	
LOW	HIGH	VERY HIGH
eggs		
fresh eggs		
frozen egg		
white mix		
dry pavlova		
mix (no		
preservative)		
soy products		
soymilks	soymilks with raw sugar	soy sauce, miso
soy yoghurt,	(**S**), coldpressed oil (**S**),	tempeh, tamari **AG**
no annatto	or unlisted anti-	
160b	oxidants, see p. 00.	
tofu, firm or		
smooth		
vanilla soy		
icecream		
others		
oatmilk	as above	
ricemilk		
Nuttelex		
dairy–free		
margarine		

Egg substitutes like Orgran Egg-like are failsafe.

Drinks

DRINK	AVOID S = salicylates A = amines G = glutamates		
LOW	MODERATE	HIGH	VERY HIGH
water, spring water	commercial pear juice (contains peel) **S**	most fruit juices **S**	orange juice **SA** tomato juice **SAG** vegetable juice **SAG**
soda water			
magic cordial, p. 246			
	lemonade, bottled, no preservatives tonic water, bottled, no preservatives **SA**		cordials, soft drinks, fruit flavoured drinks and mineral waters **S** cola (Coke, Pepsi etc) **SA**
plain milk (cow, goat, sheep), malted milk powder			chocolate milk **A** other flavoured milk **S** cocoa **A** chocolate flavoured drinks (Milo, Quik etc) **A**
tea and coffee			
decaffeinated coffee	coffee, coffee substitutes **S**		tea **S**
carob powder	decaf tea **S** herbal tea **S**		peppermint tea **S**

Choose from the low column during your elimination diet. Water is the best drink. If you don't like the taste, try a filter. Avoid sports drinks and any other drink with colours, flavours, preservatives. Failsafe lemonade, see see *Failsafe Cookbook*, is strictly limited to 150 ml per week (less than one glass) because of SA in the lemon juice flavour. You might need to limit decaf to 2 cups per day. With carob powder, be careful, many people complain about reactions to a darker, more bitter variety.

Alcohol

DRINK	AVOID S = salicylates A = amines G = glutamates		
LOW **alcohol** gin vodka whisky	MODERATE	HIGH	VERY HIGH sake **A** beer **SA** cider **SA** brandy **SAG** liqueur **SAG** port **SAG** rum **SAG** sherry **SAG** wine **SAG**

Oils, nuts, snacks

EAT	AVOID S = salicylates A = amines G = glutamates		
LOW	MODERATE	HIGH	VERY HIGH
oils	almond S	coconut oil SA	
canola, soy,	corn oil S	copha SA	
safflower, or	peanut oil S	olive oil SA	
sunflower oil		sesame oil SA	
cottonseed		walnut oil SA	
margarine		flaxseed S	
from oils above		linseed S	
snacks			
cashews (raw)	tacos S	brazil nuts SA	almonds SA
plain potato	corn chips S	cashews,	
crisps, no		roasted SA	fruit
antioxidants		coconut SA	flavours SA
pretzels		hazelnuts SA	honey
		macadamia SA	flavours S
		peanuts SA	muesli bars SA
		pecans SA	spicy
		pinenuts SA	flavours SAG
		pistachio SA	cheese
		pumpkin	flavours AG
		seeds SA	
		sesame	
		seeds SA	
		sunflower	
		seeds SA	
		walnuts SA	

Choose from the low column during your elimination diet. Refined reduces food chemicals. Refining reduces salicylates. Avoid cold-pressed oils (**S**) except for soy. Avoid oils, margarines and products containing oils with antioxidants 310–312 and 319–321. Margarine with colour 160a is failsafe, not 160b or artificial colours. Avoid commercial salad dressings and mayonnaise. Avoid snack food with colours, flavours, flavour enhancers, preservatives and antioxidants, above. Raw cashews are limited to 10 per day. Poppyseeds are failsafe. Avoid flavoured chips, hot chips and fries (antioxidants, sulphites). See snack suggestions p. 243.

Flavourings

EAT	AVOID S = salicylates A = amines G = glutamates		
LOW	MODERATE	HIGH	VERY HIGH
salt (sea, rock)			flavoured
			salts **SAG**
chives		fresh herbs **S**	HVP, HPP,
garlic		dried herbs **S**	TVP **AG**
shallots		spices **S**	meat
parsley			extracts **AG**
poppyseeds			soy paste **AG**
			soy sauce **AG**
saffron			
			tandoori **SA**
citric acid	malt vinegar **A**		vinegar except
			malt **SA**
vanilla			
(2 drops/day)			gravies,
			homemade **A**
			or premix **SAG**
			pastes (fish,
			meat and
			tomato) **SAG**
			sauces **SAG**
			meat
			marinades
			SAG
			tomato sauce,
			puree **SAG**
			stock cubes
			SAG
			yeast extracts
			like Vegemite
			SAG

Avoid flavoured salts like garlic, ham seasoning, etc. Avoid HVP (hydro-lysed vegetable protein), HPP (hydrolysed plant protein), TVP (textured vegetable protein). Avoid all fresh and dried herbs (including herbal medicines) and spices including allspice, aniseed, bayleaf, cardamom, carraway, cayenne, chili, cinnamon, cloves, coriander, cumin, curry, dill, five spice, garam marsala, ginger, mace, mint, mixed herbs, mustard, nutmeg, oregano, paprika, pepper, pimiento, rosemary, sage, tarragon, turmeric. Use a small amount of parsley for colour only.

Sweets, spreads, cooking ingredients

EAT	AVOID S = salicylates A = amines	
	G = glutamates	
LOW	MODERATE	VERY HIGH
sugars		
sugar (white, brown,	raw sugar S	honey S
icing or caster)	molasses S	
golden syrup	treacle S	liquorice S
maple syrup		mint–flavoured
malt extract		sweets S
		peppermints S
sweets, see below		chewing gum S
	chocolate (white) A	fruit flavoured
spreads		sweets S
caramel topping		chocolate (brown) A
p. 234		cocoa A
pear jam, ketchup,		
p. 256, 257		jams, jellies SA
magic spread,		lemon butter SA
cashew paste, raw,		peanut butter SA
see Cookbook		cashew paste
		roasted SA
baking aids		Nutella SA
baking powder		Yeast extracts,
bicarbonate of soda		Vegemite, Marmite,
(500)		Promite SAG
citric acid (330)		
cream of tartar (334)		
gelatine (remove		
sulphur dioxide by		
boiling)		
bakers yeast		
Jamsetta		

Avoid maple flavoured syrup (preservatives). Sweets must be from permitted ingredients (avoid colours, preservatives, added flavour except vanilla) see Cookbook: carob, caramels, toffees, butterscotch, white marshmallows, milk-based sweets, asthmatics be careful of sulphites in glucose syrup and gelatine based sweets. Raw cashew nut paste limited to 2 tsp/day. Jamsetta is for jam-making: sugar, citric acid, pectin. Avoid fruit-flavoured sweets and ices. Make home-cooking from permitted ingredients (biscuits, cakes, muffins, scones, pancakes, pikelets). Avoid commercial products with colours, preservatives, added flavours), see shopping list p. 232.

Pharmaceuticals

ALLOWED	AVOID
medications	medications which are not essential
essential prescription medications (antibiotics, antihistamines, asthma medications etc)	
	coloured tablets, capsules syrups, solutions, liquids with colour, flavour, preservatives; colour–free children's syrups with flavours, preservatives; cough syrups, lozenges
white tablets	
capsules (powdered contents)	
antacid tablets and powders (no colours or flavours)	
	salicylates in: aspirin preparations, non–steroidal anti–inflammatory drugs, eucalyptus oil, menthol, oil of wintergreen (Vicks Vaporub, Deep Heat etc).
pain relief: paracetamol, codeine (Panadol, Panadeine), acetaminophen	
local anaesthetic (no preservative)	
supplements	
vitamins (no PABA, colours, flavours)	liquid, flavoured, chewable, or megadose vitamins, supplements.
calcium supplements (no colours, flavour)	herbal remedies
iron supplements (no colour, flavour)	essential oils, aromatherapy, incense

Prescribed medications are not necessarily failsafe, but if they are essential you must put up with the consequences. For some coloured tablets, you can wash off the coloured coating. Open coloured capsules, empty powdered contents on to a saucer and mix with syrup, see p. 84. Use salt or soda bicarbonate as a toothpaste substitute. Many people become more sensitive to strong smells for a few months when starting an elimination diet.

Toiletries

ALLOWED	AVOID
toothpaste (no colour, flavour, p. 275)	colours, flavours, mouthwashes
soaps, shampoos, conditioners, moisturisers (light or unscented)	strongly perfumed products perfumes after shave lotion
deodorants (roll–on or stick)	aerosol deodorants or hairspray
sunscreen without PABA	sunscreen with PABA
laundry detergents, soap powders (unscented, no enzymes, p. 239)	fabric conditioners, washing and ironing sprays

AVOID THESE ADDITIVES

Artificial colours
102 tartrazine
104 quinoline yellow
110 sunset yellow
122 carmoisine
123 amaranth
124 ponceau
127 erythrosine
129 allura red
132 indigotine
133 brilliant blue
142 food green
143 fast green
151 brilliant black
155 chocolate brown

Natural colour
160b annatto

Preservatives
200–203 sorbic acid and sorbates
210–213 benzoic acid and banzoates
220–228 sulphur dioxide and sulphites
280–283 propionic acid and proprionates
249–252 nitrates, nitrites

Antioxidants
310–312 gallates
319 TBHQ
320 BHA
321 BHT

Flavour enhancers
620–625 Glutamates, MSG, HVP, HPP
627 Disodium guanylate
631 Disodium inosinate
635 Ribonucleotides

Shopping list

Read ingredient labels. Ingredients change constantly. For more details and updates see my website www.fedupwithfood additives.info.

Dairy-free, wheat-free and gluten-free suggestions are at the end of the list.

Very sensitive people will react to some of the foods on this list.

FRESH VEGETABLES

Potatoes (large white or dirty brown), swedes

Brussels sprouts, cabbage, red cabbage

Green beans (fresh, dried if no preservative, frozen)

Celery, parsley, iceberg lettuce

Chokoes

Leeks, garlic, shallots, chives

Canned or dried lentils and beans e.g. kidney or butter beans (not broad beans)

Mungbean sprouts, bamboo shoots

FROZEN VEGETABLES

Green beans, Brussels sprouts, diced swede, celery cuts, lima beans, butter beans

CANNED VEGETABLES

Green beans, lima beans, soy beans, red kidney beans, butter beans, borlotti beans, chick peas, three bean mix, four bean mix, bean sprouts (Trident), bamboo shoots (Changs)

DRIED VEGETABLES

Split peas (yellow or green), chick peas, besan flour, lentils (red, brown, green), borlotti beans, soy beans, canellini beans, lima beans, haricot beans, black eye beans, red kidney beans

FRUIT

Pears, peeled, ripe, soft and juicy

Pears canned in light syrup *not juice*

baby pear puree (Heinz, Gerber)

limit 2 whole pears/day but this is too much for the very sensitive

PASTA, NOODLES, FLOUR, RICE

Wheat flour (bleached, unbleached, wholemeal, plain, self-raising), wheaten cornflour

Pasta, spaghetti, durum wheat, barley, rye (no colour, flavour, fillings)

Noodles, uncoloured Asian-style instant (no flavour sachet, Trident, Changs)

Couscous

Rice noodles

Rice, white, brown or gold but not flavoured like basmati or jasmine

Barley, flour, unpearled, pearl, flakes

Wheat, barley, oat or rice bran

Wheatgerm

Semolina

BREAD

No preservative 280–283, no whey powder, no vinegar, no fruit, no honey, no 223, 319, 320. Plain or poppyseed, Brumby's plain breads—loaves, rolls, French bread; Franklins Big Fresh, Country Life Bakery, Demeter, Woolworth's store baked preservative-free (check label and be careful, sometimes local bakers use the wrong premix), Mountain bread, Moores, Naturis, Dallas, Jakks. Flat bread: Fielders Pocket, Sunray Pita, Long Life Pita, Lavash, Woolworth's instore. Bagels (Sara Lee, Jakks), Brumby's iced finger buns (order with white icing, no coconut or topping). Other brands, read labels. Laucke's breadmaker premix.

BREAKFAST CEREALS

Wheat cereals Many brands such as Kellogg's Allbran, Ready Wheats, Puffed Wheat, Special K, check ingredient labels, some people do not tolerate wholegrain wheat products

Oat cereals Plain, Crunchy oat bran, Oat bran, Uncle Toby's Crunchy Oat Flakes, Bubbles, Rolled Oats, regular and quick cook

Rice cereal Kellogg's Rice Bubbles, Rice Pops, Sanitarium Ricies, Uncle Toby's Rice Crispies

Wheat pancakes, many brands are failsafe, e.g. White Wings Shaker Pancakes, White Wings Panjacks

SWEETENERS, TOPPINGS, SPREADS

White sugar, caster sugar, pure icing sugar, brown sugar (not raw sugar), golden syrup, maple syrup (pure, e.g. Camp,

Norganic), Malt extract
e.g. Saunders, Rice syrup,
rice malt syrup, pear jam,
home-made with Jamsetta,
or Birgit's pear jam (see
website), caramel dessert
topping—Windsor Farm,
Nestle Caramel Top 'n'
Fill

HEALTHFOOD SECTION
Some people react to carob
Carob powder (not from
Turkey), carob buttons, no
added flavour, cashew nuts
(raw, limited), cashew nut
paste (raw, *not* lightly
roasted)

CAKES, MUFFINS, BISCUITS
May contain egg and milk
Sara Lee all-purpose pound
cake, self-saucing sponge
(Big Sister Butterscotch,
Big Sister Golden),
Defiance instant success
multi purpose Baking Mix,
Defiance Hot Cake Mix,
White Wings Biscuit Base,
Betty Crocker Bisquick

PASTRY
May contain milk, soy, egg
Pampas Puff Pastry, Pampas
filo pastry, Greens Pastry
mix, Spring Roll Pastry
(TYJ, Trangs, Pampas)

BISCUITS
*Note: any biscuit containing
vegetable oil may also
contain antioxidant
(319–321) despite the
label. The reaction is dose
related—the more you eat,
the more likely you are to
react. The oil in Arnott's
biscuits is now failsafe.*
Arnotts original water
crackers, wholemeal Sao,
Sao, Salada, Saltine,
Vitaweet, Rice cakes
(plain or with buckwheat,
thick are unlimited, thin
may contain antioxidants
in vegetable oil, limited),
Shortbreads (e.g.
Glengarry) made from
flour, butter and sugar,
Milk Coffee Biscuits,
Milk Arrowroots

MEAT
*Use the day you buy or freeze
and eat within 4 weeks.*
Beef, e.g. preservative-free
mince, steak, chops, roast
beef, lamb e.g. chops, leg
of lamb, lamb steak, veal,
sausages specially made
with fresh meat, rice flour,
sea salt, shallots and/or
garlic, sausages from
Colvic Focus Foods

CHICKEN

It is not enough to avoid the skin and stuffing on a seasoned, stuffed chicken.

Whole fresh, frozen or rotisserie chicken (no skin, definitely no seasoning, stuffing, or self-basting), chicken fillets, thighs, pieces (no skin, no marinade)

FISH

Cook within 12 hours of capture or freeze and use within 2 weeks.

Fresh (not frozen or canned) white fish (e.g. snapper, barramundi, whiting, not salmon, tuna), crab, lobster, oysters, calamari, scallops but not prawns

EGGS

Fresh eggs, preferably free range, frozen egg white mix (Good Food, Just white, Yolk free), Pavlova mix if additive-free (Greens Ezi-pav, Pavlova magic)

EGG REPLACER

Egglike (Country Harvest), Orgran egg replacer, Nutricia

DAIRY FOODS
(IF DAIRY IS PERMITTED)

Thickeners in yoghurt, icecream and thickened cream may contain small amounts of gluten.

Milk: fresh, plain, full cream, skim, buttermilk, UHT, sweetened condensed, powdered, evaporated, and reduced lactose (Balance).

Yoghurt: no preservatives, no 160b; plain *(beware of very sharp taste for the extra sensitive, especially amine responders)*; vanilla *(some people will react to added flavour especially if eaten frequently)*; Vaalia Ski, Nestle Activ LC1, Fruche French Vanilla, Yoplait Petit Miam Vanilla Surprise fromage frais (not yoghurt).

Fresh white cheeses like: Philadelphia cream cheese, Ricotta (Perfection cheeses, Avanti, Paesanella, Norco, La Deliziosa, United Dairies, No Frills), Cottage cheese (no preservative—Jalna, Avanti)

Icecream: Peters Original Vanilla icecream, Norco Natural, Pauls, No Frills, Homebrand, MasterMaid,

Farmland, Woolworths Traditional

Ricecream Vanilla rice cream/creamed rice dessert (Jacaranda)

Cream: fresh, light, regular, rich, sour, canned, thickened, UHT

Butter: salted and unsalted (no 160b), Dairy soft, Dairy blend, Softgold, (not Country gold), Ghee

Margarine with milk: *no sorbate 200–203, 160b annatto colour; note that 160a carotene is OK.* Meadowlea (check label), Golden Pastures, Mrs McGregors, No Frills, No Name Savings Eta 5-Star Canola, Gold'n Canola (not the Lifestyle)

Non-dairy: Nuttelex margarine, Soymilk; calcium fortified, unflavoured (avoid cold-pressed oil, raw sugar, evaporated cane juice, antioxidants 319–321 e.g. SoyLife); if gluten free avoid malt—Sanitarium, So Good soymilk (UHT, not fresh), Soy yoghurt e.g. Soygurt, Soy cream cheese (King Land), Soy custard, Soy life (contains gluten), Tofu e.g. King Land Silken Tofu, Vanilla soy icecream e.g. Fruccio, Rice milk, calcium fortified, unfortified, Oatmilk

OILS

Canola oil, safflower, sunflower or soy oil, not cold pressed (except for soy), no antioxidants (310–321). In Australia, nearly all brands are failsafe, e.g. Becel, Crisco, Eta, Meadowlea, Sunola, Sunbeam. In New Zealand, only Ideal sunflower oil.

DRINKS

Water, filtered water, soda water (commercial or home made), spring water, plain mineral water, tonic water (unpreserved, e.g. Schweppes tonic water)

Milk, malted milk, soymilk

Decaffeinated coffee (instant, e.g. Nescafe or ground e.g. Lavazzo)

Soyaccino (Sanitarium)

Carob powder—not from Turkey

Unpreserved lemonade (7UP, some Schweppes, 150 ml/week)

Home-made magic cordial (buy citric acid)

Home-made pear 'juice'—
dilute syrup or fresh pears
with water or soda water—
not suitable for the very
sensitive

Gin, vodka, whisky

HOME COOKING

Salt (sea salt or rock salt),
salt substitutes e.g. Greens
Lo salt, baking powder
(Wards is gluten free),
bicarbonate of soda, citric
acid, cream of tartar,
tartaric acid, gelatine
(boil before use to remove
sulphites), vanilla essence
(natural or artificial—
limited, some people will
react to either), bakers
yeast (fresh or dried),
poppyseeds (not other
seeds), chives, garlic—
powder, granules, flakes
(not paste or in oil because
of the antioxidants not
listed on the label), saffron
powder or threads (not
artificially coloured
powder)

SNACKS

Kettle plain chips, Colvan
plain chips, Planters
classic Kettle cooked
plain salted, pretzels (e.g.
Parkers), Raw cashew nuts
(limit 10 per day), plain
pappadums (e.g. Pataks)

SWEETS AND TREATS

*Asthmatics should be careful
of any product that
contains glucose syrup or
gelatine. Be careful of any
product that contains
'flavours'. Many people
fail because they eat
products from this list every
day. Regard these as treats
and preferably <u>avoid them
during the elimination diet</u>.
Eat them as treats only
when you have improved.*

Icecream cones (The Natural
icecream cone), Pauls
dessert whip (some people
will react to flavour),
Peters microfreeze vanilla
malt thickshake (ditto),
malted milk powder
(Nestle, Horlicks)

Flavoured milk drinks—
Classic vanilla malt, Good
One carob (both limited),
Custard (Pauls, Ideal dairy
natural vanilla, Soy Life)

*Peter's Lemonade icypoles
are now not permitted, the
recipe has changed*

Marshmallows (Pascalls
Vanilla, limit 4/day)

Caramels (e.g. Allen's jersey
caramels, limited)

Butterscotch (no colours or artificial flavours so unlimited, e.g. Darrell Lea or Callard and Bowser Butterscotch but not toffee)

Toffee and butter candy (e.g. Allens McIntosh butter candy, not caramels)

Honeycomb sweets (by Darrell Lea, like the inside of Violet Crumble Bars)

Milk-based lollies such as Allen's Milk Shake lollies and Moo Choos but beware of the cumulative effects of artificial flavours and milk

Home-made plain toffees, caramels, butterscotch, caramel fudge

Only for the less sensitive . . . (I do not recommend these)

White jelly beans (limit 4/day, Darrell Lea are the only preservative-free white jelly beans, but many people react to the lemon juice, beware)

Kellogg's Rice Bubble treats, plain (definitely not for everyone!)

WHEAT FREE

Wheat and preservative-free rye bread e.g. Country Life

Rye bread, rye crisps e.g. Ryvita, Kavli, rye flour, use also gluten free brands

GLUTEN FREE

Rice, brown or white (not Jasmine, basmati, wild), rice bran, rice flour, rice noodles, vermicelli, rice pasta e.g. Orgran rice-soya garlic and parsley pasta, puffed rice cereals e.g. Happy Human Puffed Rice, Nutra life, rolled rice flakes

Millet (hulled, unhulled, flour, flakes, meal, puffed)

Buckwheat (raw, roasted, cracked, flour), buckwheat pasta, buckwheat puffs, buckwheat pancake mix (Orgran)

Amaranth puffed breakfast cereal and quinoa flour

Sago and tapioca flour and balls, arrowroot flour

Potato flour or starch, fresh potato gnocchi (Guzzi's)

Cornflour (maize not wheaten, e.g. White Wings)

Soy flour, rolled soy flakes, grits, pasta

Psyllium hulls, besan (chick pea) flour, sorghum

Xanthan gum and guar gum

BAKING MIX OR FLOUR

Gluten free, wheat free multi-purpose baking mix (many including Country Harvest, Orgran, F G Roberts)

Gluten Free Bread: *Check for milk, soy, preservative, vinegar, honey, fruit, seeds*

RR Friendly Bakery, Landsell Cottage premix, Pauls Allergy Bakery, see details on my website, under product updates

In NZ, Dovedale GF yeast-free rice bread

GF Biscuits

Rice cakes, thick, plain, with millet, with buckwheat, Carob Rice Cakes (Freedom Foods, Naturally Good), Rice Cookies (Orgran)

GF Pastry

May contain milk, soy, egg

Pizza and Pastry mix (Orgran), Rice paper, a gluten-free pastry substitute in Chinese shops

Ricecrumbs

Orgran, Casalare

TOILETRIES AND MEDICATIONS

Toothpaste, unflavoured, uncoloured (e.g. Soul Pattinson's Plain)

Soap, uncoloured, low-perfume (e.g. Sunlight, Simple, Imperial Leather, no bubble bath)

Shampoo/conditioner (Pears Natural or bulk perfume-free in Health Food stores)

Deodorant: low-perfume roll-on deodorant

Moisturiser: sorbolene, Ego and Demraveen ranges, also sunscreen

Washing powder, no perfume, no enzymes, e.g. Planet Ark, Lux, Omo-sensitive, Amway

Toilet paper, plain, uncoloured, unperfumed

Multivitamins: Macro Multi M, Amcal One-a day

Calcium: Caltrate (plain) from pharmacies.

Read labels: ingredients change!

22 Failsafe recipes

Failsafe eating is easy for a motivated adult. It is more of a challenge with a difficult child. The suggestions below are only an example.

A SAMPLE DAY

Breakfast: Rice Bubbles or rolled oats with milk • fresh or canned pear • toast (preservative–free) with margarine and pear jam.

Lunch: 1 or 2 sandwiches (preservative free bread): cold home–cooked roast chicken or cream cheese with lettuce, celery, mung sprouts.

Dinner: Grilled or panfried lamb, beef, chicken or fish with mashed potato, green beans and Brussels sprouts • or pasta with chicken and cream cheese topping • or failsafe burgers • or failsafe sausages • home–made chicken schnitzel and chips • icecream with canned pears.

Snacks: Pear • buttered crackers or rice cakes • yoghurt • raw cashew nuts • hard boiled eggs • home made or commercial plain sweet biscuits.

Drinks: Decaf coffee, milk, soymilk, water or permitted alcoholic drinks (adults only).

Each family has to find their own way. This section will give you ideas about how to adapt your present meals using failsafe ingredients. There are some recipes here and heaps more in my *Failsafe Cookbook*.

Some failsafe substitutes

alcohol	gin, vodka, whisky
baked beans	canned butter beans
biscuits	shortbreads, commercial biscuits p. 234, home-made p. 255
bread	preservative-free p. 233, rice cakes, low-fat crackers
breadcrumbs	rice crumbs or home-made breadcrumbs
brown sugar	light brown sugar, not dark and coloured with molasses
burgers	home-made p. 249
butter	pure butter, dairy blend, margarine see p. 257
cakes	home made p. 254 or commercial no additives, p. 234
cheese	white cheeses, p. 223, soycheese with 160a not 160b
chicken nuggets	home-made, p. 249
chocolate	use carob instead of chocolate, cocoa, Milo
cooking oil	p. 256
cordial	p. 246
croissants	no colours, preservatives, antioxidants, whey powder
crumb mix	see breadcrumbs
dried fruit	soft, ripe pears dried in a home dehydrator (limited)
fish fingers	home-made, p. 249
'flavours'	enjoy the flavour of fresh, natural, high quality ingredients
fries	homemade, p. 250, failsafe potato crisps, p. 237
ginger	(in gingerbread) brown sugar, see *Failsafe Cookbook*
gluten-free	see pp. 238–39
icypoles	home-made, p. 246
jam	p. 256, or see website
juice	water, home-made icypoles p. 246, magic cordial p. 246
honey	golden syrup, maple syrup, rice malt
KFC	HFC, see the *Failsafe Cookbook*
lemon juice	'citric' lemon juice p. 258
margarine	p. 257
milk	if dairy free: soymilk, ricemilk, oatmilk
noodles	uncoloured noodles, no flavour sachet
pasta topping	p. 252

peanut butter	home-made cashew paste
pizza	home-made, p. 251
salt	use for flavour—failsafe eating is naturally low in salt
soft drinks	see p. 225
soy sauce	golden syrup
tomato sauce	pear ketchup, pear puree, mayo, leek sauce, all pp. 256–58
toothpaste	plain, unflavoured toothpaste p. 239 or salt
sweets	toffees, caramels, butterscotch, others, p. 255
Vegemite	plain buttered toast
vitamins	Macro Multi M or Amcal One-a-day, p. 239

Breakfasts are easy

You can choose from the following: cereal—rolled oats with brown sugar, commercial cereals such as Rice Bubbles, (see shopping list p. 232) • eggs, chops • toast with butter, golden syrup or home-made pear jam • pancakes, home-made or commercial with butter or margarine and pure maple syrup • fruit: pear, fresh or canned in syrup • yoghurt: mild natural or vanilla, no annatto (160b) • dairy free: soy, rice or oat milk • gluten-free: puffed rice, puffed amaranth, boiled rice, rice cakes, gluten free toast, soymilk with no malt • drinks: decaf coffee, hot carob, milk, water.

Lunches and snacks

'Breakfast is easy, dinner is easy, it's the lunches and snacks I find hard on this diet'—Failsafe parent

SANDWICH SUGGESTIONS

Use preservative-free bread and rolls or rice cakes with failsafe butter or margarine (p. 257) • home-cooked fresh or frozen roast chicken, lamb and beef with salt, lettuce, chopped shallots, mung bean sprouts, parsley or celery • rissoles, sausages, sliced hard-boiled egg • butter beans • cream cheese, soy cream cheese, preservative-free cottage cheese, egg • hard-boiled and mixed with a little warm milk and salt • cashew paste (make your own from raw cashews, oil, salt, see *Failsafe Cookbook*) • pear jam (p. 256) • rice malt • golden syrup.

LUNCHBOX SUGGESTIONS
Sandwich (p. 242) • slice of
failsafe quiche, pizza, cold
sausage (p. 248) or rissole
(meat leftovers should be
frozen) • home-made pie
or small sausage rolls,
p. 244 (some tuckshops
will reheat them for you) •

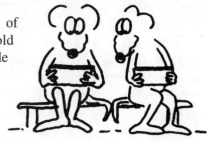

vanilla yoghurt or soy yoghurt • stick of celery • hard boiled egg
• cashew nuts, raw (limit 10 per day) • small container with
chopped canned pear • home-made treats like lunchbox muffins
(p. 254), cookies (p. 255), cake (p. 254), Sarah Lee vanilla
pound cake or plain sweet biscuits like shortbreads, see
shopping list (p. 232) • failsafe pretzels or chips, p. 237 • white
iced finger buns from Brumby's hot bread shops, you might
need to order these the day before—they can be frozen in
separate bags and used, cut in half, or sliced and buttered in
school lunchboxes • water, Soyaccino, magic cordial or soy
shake in a spring water bottle with a small amount of water
frozen in the bottom.

PRESCHOOL ALTERNATIVES TO A PLATE OF FRUIT
Fresh peeled pear • Golden or Red Delicious apple when
permitted • buttered failsafe crackers (for example, Saladas) •
pear puree icypole • home made biscuits • for baking days or
birthday parties, make a special iced birthday cake at home, cut
it into slices, wrap each piece in cling film and put in a freezer
bag with your child's name on it. Keep a few slices in the
preschool freezer.

SNACK SUGGESTIONS
As for lunchboxes, also: fresh peeled pear or canned pear (limit
2 whole pears per day) • buttered rice cakes, permitted rice
crackers, or wheat-based crackers like Saladas with failsafe
margarine or with spreads like cashew paste, cream cheese,
golden syrup or pear jam • homemade fresh bread rolls with

butter or garlic butter (p. 264) • preservative-free toast, celery sticks with cream cheese • plate of raw salad vegetables (p. 251) with dip (p. 257) • icypoles (p. 246), jelly cups, sago or custard cups, scones, pikelets and pancakes (*Failsafe Cookbook*) • some additive-free commercial croissants • toasted sandwiches or steak sandwich • home-made potato wedges • vegetable soup • egg on toast • plate of pasta with butter and salt (see p. 252) or mince topping (p. 248) • anything from the breakfast, lunch section or dinner sections • Peters Dixie cup icecreams, sweets, homemade or limited commercial • Kelloggs Rice Bubble Treats (LCMs) limited to less than 1 per week—none for some children, see p. 275.

A school looking for an additive–free pie found most contained artificial colours or annatto (160b) in the crust. All contained either MSG or hydrolysed vegetable protein (HVP) which is a form of MSG. All contained BHA (320) in fats or vegetable oils, including one pie which claimed to be additive–free.

Pies and sausage rolls

You can make your own sausage rolls from mince (flavoured with shallots, garlic, salt), form into sausage shape and place on the middle of a half sheet of Pampas pastry. Roll over, prick top.

Q. What's in a hot dog?
A. When we checked, one brand of frankfurts and saveloys contained sodium metabisulphite (223) and sodium nitrite (250). The colour in the skins weren't listed but turned out to be annatto (160b) and cochineal (120). The roll will probably contain calcium propionate (282).

Cut to required lengths. Bake 20 minutes or until cooked. Use an automatic pie-maker to make pies with failsafe mince or other fillings. See tomato sauce alternatives (p. 257), but after a while you won't miss it.

FINGER FOODS FOR BABIES AND TODDLERS
(In an allergic family, delay introduction of eggs, dairy foods, nuts and seafood usually until 12 months: your dietitian can advise you.)

rusks: bake fingers of bread or rye bread in a slow oven for 2 hours or until very hard—good for teething • pureed baby pears or stewed pear • bananas (moderate in amines, if tolerated) • fingers of steamed cooked potato, swede, celery, pumpkin, sweet potato and carrots when permitted • failsafe vegetables— steamed and mashed, formed into a finger shape or different shapes, rolled in rice crumbs (p. 239), bake in a moderate oven for 10–15 minutes or until crispy on the outside • chicken fingers—finger shaped patties of minced chicken, made up with cornflour, oats if permitted and a pinch of salt, bake for 20 minutes or panfried in a little failsafe oil for a real treat • fish fingers—flaked white fish fillets, mixed with mashed potato and dipped in cornflour, egg, rice crumbs • over 12 months, strips of egg • home baked biscuits (reduced sugar is a good idea) • mini sausage rolls (p. 244) • home made icypoles.

Drinks
Water • spring water • soda water • preservative-free tonic (e.g. Schweppes) • home-made milkshakes—from milk, soymilk or ricemilk, flavoured with carob, decaf or caramel topping (p. 234), permitted icecream • preservative-free lemonade (e.g. 7UP, some Schweppes, limited to one small glass a week because it contains salicylates and amines in lemon juice).

Magic cordial

Our grandmothers called this 'poor man's lemonade'.

1 cup sugar
1 cup water
$^1\!/_2$–1 tsp citric acid.

Place water and sugar in a 2 cup jug and heat in microwave for two minutes. Stir until sugar is dissolved. Add citric acid. Store in refrigerator. Dilute to taste with water or soda water, about 1:4.

Variations: Hot 'lemon' drink, as above, but serve hot and stir in a pinch of white Vitamin C powder before serving • **Whisky Sour**—add to whisky and soda water.

Icypoles and icecups

You will need your own icypole moulds or plastic cups. Adjust dilutions to suit individual tastes. More water makes the icypole harder, more sugar makes it softer. You can use: plain water • magic cordial, diluted • pear syrup diluted with equal quantities of water (limit 2 whole pears or equivalent per day) • baby pear puree, or canned pears, blended without syrup • yoghurt or home-made iced decaf with extra

Peters Lemonade icypoles were previously permitted once a week. The recipe has changed. There are now no failsafe commercial icypoles.

sugar.

Main meals

Vegetable soup

1 cup (half a 375 g packet) of
   red lentils—these cook much
   more quickly than brown lentils
4 cups water or home-made
   chicken stock (p. 000)
1 tbsp failsafe oil
1 cup celery, chopped
1 cup leeks or shallots, sliced
2 potatoes, peeled and cubed or
   one potato, one swede
3 cups sliced cabbage
6 Brussels sprouts, halved
1 cup frozen green peas
   (moderate, use only when
   you have passed your pea
   challenge, p. 170)
extra water

Rinse lentils well. Cover lentils with water or stock and bring to the boil. In a separate saucepan, sauté celery and leeks and add to lentils. Prepare and add remaining vegetables. Add extra water until vegetables are just covered. Reduce heat and simmer gently until cooked, about 40 minutes. Blend or mash. Serves 8.

Commercial soups usually contain MSG and may contain sulphites in the vegetables. Dry packet soups can contain high levels of sulphites in the dried vegetables.

Meat (beef, lamb, veal)
SAUSAGES

Commercial sausages always contain sodium metabisulphite (223) unless labelled preservative-free. You can ask your butcher to make failsafe sausages for you, see below. A growing number of butchers are selling frozen failsafe sausages (see website). Check ingredients, however. Sausages labelled 'preservative and gluten-free' are not failsafe because they usually contain herbs and spices and may contain MSG.

A recipe for your butcher
For 10 kg sausages

650 g brown rice flour
  (2 kg for 30 kg)

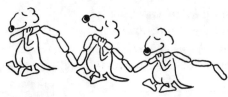

3 leeks (10 leeks for
  30 kg)
3 cloves garlic or less
  (10 for 30 kg)
$\frac{1}{2}$ cup sea salt ($1\frac{1}{2}$ cups for 30 kg)
make up to 10 kg with fresh minced beef or chicken

Failsafe mince

Because this recipe does not disguise the flavour of the meat with MSG and strongly flavoured sauces, the mince needs to be fresh and good quality. If you can't find good mince, ask your butcher to prepare minced topside steak for you. Ask your butcher: 'Does this mince contain preservatives? I really need to know.'

500 g preservative-free low fat
  beef or lamb mince
2 shallots or 1 leek, finely
  chopped
1 clove or more garlic, crushed
1 tbsp failsafe oil (p. 256)
sea salt to taste
1 tsp chopped parsley
2 tbsp cornflour dissolved in
  2 cups of water or home-made
  chicken stock (p. 259)

In a heavy–based frypan or large saucepan stirfry chopped shallots and garlic in failsafe oil, remove from heat. Add mince to pan, stir until cooked. Drain fat if necessary. Add shallots, garlic, parsley, sea–salt and cornflour mixture, stir until thickened. Serve on mashed potato, pasta, noodles, rice, cous cous, toast, pizza and in jaffles and pies. Suitable to make a double batch and freeze in small containers if used within four weeks.

Burgers

'Make mince patties with egg, garlic, finely chopped leek, salt, sprinkle of citric acid. Serve on rolls or toast with lettuce, sprouts, sometimes an extra fried egg. Non-failsafe family members can add whatever they like—beetroot, tomato, sauce, etc, which means everyone is happy'—reader, Sydney

---

Browning meat, charring, or grilling will increase amine content. It is best to aim for medium rare. Extremely sensitive amine responders may need to steam or microwave their meat. Delicious tasting meat juices and gravy made from meat juices are high in amines, see p. 222. Marinades must be made of failsafe ingredients. Any commercial marinade, sauce or gravy is very high in salicylates, amines and MSG.

Chicken schnitzel

Kids love crumbed food which can ease the pain of avoiding takeaways. You can also use this method for fish, crumbed cutlets and veal schnitzel. These are good hot or cold and can be used in lunchboxes.

500 g chicken breasts, cut into
  thin slices
flour or gluten-free flour
$^1/_2$ tsp salt
1 egg, beaten
home-made bread crumbs or
  rice crumbs
failsafe oil (p. 256) for frying

Cut chicken into thin slices or nugget shapes. Season flour with salt, then coat chicken slices. Dip into beaten egg and cover with crumbs. Fry gently in shallow oil until golden brown on both sides. Drain on paper towels. Garnish with parsley and serve with mashed potato, vegetables and citric lemon juice (p. 258).

Commercial breadcrumbs all contain preservative (282) and some contain HVP (MSG). Use rice crumbs instead.

Andra's quick chicken and noodles

1 tbsp failsafe oil, p. 256
1 cup each failsafe vegetables
    (e.g. leek, cabbage, green
    beans, carrots if permitted)
1 chicken breast fillet, cut into
    strips
extra oil
4 cups water
1 cup homemade chicken stock
    p. 259) or water
2 packets (250 gm each) of
    instant noodles, rice or wheat,
    e.g. Fantastic rice noodles
1 tsp salt

Heat oil in a very large pot, saute vegetables. Remove from pan. Add extra oil and saute chicken strips until light brown. Add vegetables to pan and add liquid. Arrange noodles over vegetables, add salt and put lid on pot. Cook for 6–8 minutes, stirring occasionally. For very sensitive amine responders, you can omit chicken stock, remove chicken after sautéeing and add at the end, reheating for a few minutes.

TWO–MINUTE NOODLES
Choose colour–free noodles such as *Fantastic* and avoid flavour sachets which are high in MSG. See topping suggestions (p. 252).

Oven fries

large white potatoes, peeled
    thickly
failsafe oil or spray (p. 256)
sea salt

Cut potatoes into thick chip shapes and microwave until nearly soft. Coat in failsafe oil by putting them in a plastic bag with the oil and gently rolling around, or spray with oil. Spread in a single layer on an oven tray. Bake for 20–25 minutes at 180°C. Serve sprinkled with salt. Oiled, unbaked chips can be frozen for later use.

Commercial hot chips and fries may have been dipped in suphites. They are almost always cooked in oil containing at least one harmful antioxidant. They may also contain colours like 160b.

Mum's mash: getting vegetables into children

Start with mashed potato with butter, milk and salt. Very slowly, add small but increasing amounts of swedes, Brussels sprouts and chokos. You can also hide vegetables in mince dishes.

SALADS

For failsafe salad vegetables you will have to make do with celery, iceberg lettuce, mung bean sprouts, red or green cabbage, raw swede sticks, raw choko sticks, cold cooked green beans, dried beans such as kidney or butter beans. With these, you can do a tossed salad, coleslaw, plate of failsafe vegetables or a bean and pasta salad with cooked green beans. See p. 257 for dressing substitutes. If you fail your salicylate challenge you will probably have an allowance of moderate vegetables including asparagus, beetroot, carrot, Chinese greens, lettuce other than iceberg, snow peas and snow pea sprouts if tolerated.

PIZZA

You can make your own failsafe pizzas especially if you have a breadmaker for the dough. Some failsafe toppings: **garlic meat topping**: make the failsafe mince on p. 248 with extra garlic • **cheese**: spread pizza base thickly with preservative-free cream cheese. If you do not react to amines and dairy, you can sprinkle over grated mozzarella cheese • **vegetarian**: process 2 tins of partially drained red kidney beans with garlic to form a smooth paste • **chicken topping**: spread base with thick layer of cream cheese, sprinkle over chopped cooked chicken or leftover roast, sliced canned pear, and a sprinkle of finely chopped parsley.

Commercial garlic bread can contain calcium propionate (282) in the bread, colours (102, 110 or 160b), preservatives (200, 202) and antioxidants (319, 320, 321) in the garlic margarine. Make your own, see the *Failsafe Cookbook*.

PASTA

Serve any type of pasta—from twists to spaghetti—with failsafe toppings ranging from butter, garlic and salt, to garlic failsafe mince to the recipe below.

Chicken and cream cheese sauce

$^1/_2$ cup water
1 tsp parsley, finely chopped
1 tbsp shallots, finely chopped
sea salt to taste
2 tbsp cream cheese or soy cream cheese
200 g chopped, cooked chicken

Add parsley and shallots to water. Microwave on high for one minute. Stir in cream cheese. Stir in chicken. Pour over pasta. Serve with green beans. Serves two.

Fresh garlic is safest. Garlic salt might contain MSG and if crushed garlic contains vegetable oil it will probably contain unlabelled antioxidants like BHA (320).

Other main meal suggestions: panfried or grilled fish, chicken, chops or steak; roast chicken, beef or lamb (no gravy, see alternatives p. 257–58); omelettes, quiche, potato and egg or cream oven bakes; and lasagne—see recipes and more suggestions in the *Failsafe Cookbook*.

Something sweet

People who are avoiding additives but not salicylates and amines can eat fresh fruit (except grapes) but not dried fruit like apricots and coconut which contain sulphur dioxide. There are recipes for desserts from family dinners with pancakes, pear crumble to cheesecakes, pavlovas and special occasion desserts in the *Failsafe Cookbook*.

ICE CREAM

There are failsafe commercial dairy and non-dairy vanilla ice creams, see p. 235, avoid yellow colour, either artificial or annatto (160b). Commercial ice cream toppings contain preservatives and colours. Use pure maple syrup or caramel topping (p. 234).

'Lemon' meringue pie

This dessert looks fantastic and kids love it. There are no lemons—the secret ingredient is citric acid. Boiling will drive off most suphites in gelatine, but this recipe may not be suitable for extra-sensitive asthmatics.

Base

3 tbsp failsafe butter or margarine, p. 257

2 tbsp brown sugar

1 cup self raising flour (or gluten-free self raising flour), sifted

water if required

Filling

250 ml water

8 tbsp sugar

2 tsp citric acid

250 ml water, extra

5 tbsp cornflour

1 tsp gelatine

1 tbsp failsafe butter

3 egg yolks

Meringue

3 egg whites

$1/2$ cup caster sugar

pinch salt

1 tsp cornflour

Preheat oven to 180°C. To make base, beat butter and sugar together and stir in flour until it forms a ball. Add a little water if necessary. Spread evenly by hand in a 24 cm pie dish. Bake for 15 minutes and cool. Combine water, sugar and citric acid in a saucepan and bring to the boil. Reduce heat. Combine extra water, cornflour and gelatine, stir until smooth and add to the boiling syrup, stirring vigorously until thickened. Stir in butter and egg yolks. Cool a little and pour into pie crust. For meringue topping, beat eggs to a soft peak. Add sugar, salt and cornflour a little at a time, beating until glossy. Bake for 10 minutes or until golden. Note: this recipe doubled fits into a lamington tin, or standard American 13" × 9" baking pan.

Margie's Lunchbox muffins

1¹/₂ cups self-raising flour
¹/₂ cup sugar or brown sugar
1 egg, lightly beaten
³/₄ cup milk or soymilk
¹/₄ cup failsafe oil (p. 256)
¹/₂ cup chopped pears (optional)

Sift flour into a bowl and add remaining ingredients, stirring with a fork until mixed. Lightly grease a 12 cup muffin pan with failsafe margarine or brush with failsafe oil and use an icecream scoop or spoon to three–quarter fill cups. Bake at 180°C for 15–20 minutes. For a treat, ice with white icing or add flavour–free carob buttons. These are equally good with gluten–free flour.

Basic plain cake

125 g failsafe butter or margarine
   (p. 257)
125 g sugar
2 eggs, well beaten
250 g self-raising flour or
   gluten-free flour (p. 239)
¹/₄ tsp salt
¹/₂ cup milk

Grease a cake tin. Preheat oven to 180°C. Sift flour and salt. Cream butter and sugar. Add beaten eggs gradually. Add flour and salt alternately with milk and vanilla. Put in tin and bake 40–45 minutes. Ice with white icing.

Variation: cup cakes—use paper patty cases. Makes 24. Bake for 12–15 minutes. Ice with white icing. These make a good plate to take to a party or a school fete.

Basic biscuits

125 g failsafe butter or
    margarine (p. 257)
$^1/_2$ cup sugar (caster or icing)
1 egg
1 cup self raising flour
1 cup plain flour

Preheat oven to 180°C.
Cream the butter and sugar,
add egg, mix thoroughly.
Add sifted flours and mix,
knead until smooth on a
floured surface. Roll and cut
into desired shapes. Place on
a greased tray and bake for
15–20 minutes.

Sweet treats

It is possible to make a wide range of failsafe caramels, butterscotch, honeycomb, fudge, toffees, marshmallows and milk-
based sweets (see *Failsafe Cookbook*), but nearly all
commercial confectionery contains unsuitable colours, flavours,
preservatives or antioxidants in margarines. Sulphited glucose
syrup in sweets like jelly beans and gelatine in sweets like
marshmallows are a potential problem for asthmatics. When
making your own, you can boil the gelatine to drive off sulphur
dioxide, but glucose syrup may contain well over the legal limit
of sulphites and is best avoided.

Lollipops

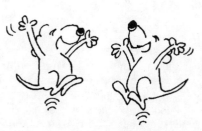

1 cup sugar
$^2/_3$ cup water
wooden sticks

Heat sugar and water in heavy-based saucepan over low heat
and stir with wooden spoon until sugar dissolves. Then bring to
the boil and simmer without stirring until a drop snaps in cold
water. Arrange rows of small sticks on oiled trays. Drop one tsp
of toffee on to pointed end of each stick. Allow to set firmly. For
a treat, put these lollipops in a small cellophane bag sealed with
a fancy sticker.

Miscellaneous

Birgit's pear jam

Pears must be soft and ripe, or your jam will contain some salicylates. Jam-making generally requires roughly equal quantities of sugar and fruit.

1 kg ripe pears, peeled and cut into small pieces (should be about 750 g)

or 2 large tins of soft pears, drained

750 g sugar

1 × 50 g packet of Jamsetta (pectin and sugar mix, available in supermarkets)

Puree pears. Put in a large saucepan and heat gently. Add sugar and Jamsetta, stirring with a wooden spoon until sugar is dissolved then bring to the boil and boil rapidly for five minutes, stirring occasionally. Allow to cool. Pour into sterilised glass jars or plastic storage containers. Store in refrigerator or freezer.

FAILSAFE OILS

Canola, safflower, sunflower and soy oils are failsafe ● cold pressed oils are not failsafe (too many salicylates) except for soy ● avoid antioxidants 310–312 and 319–321. They will be listed on the label of cooking oils if present (but not when in other products) ● in Australia, nearly all domestic cooking oils are failsafe (but not in restaurants) ● in New Zealand, nearly all cooking oils contain harmful antioxidants.

FAILSAFE MARGARINE, DAIRY BLEND
Choose margarine made with canola, sunflower, safflower or soy oils • avoid preservatives 200–203 • avoid antioxidants 310–312, 319–321 • avoid colours 102, 110, 160b but 160a is failsafe • milk–free if necessary • in Australia, there are several failsafe margarines and one failsafe dairy–free margarine, Nuttelex, which is now available in New Zealand • phone manufacturers of dairy blends to ask about antioxidants in oil.

Quick mayonnaise

400 g tin sweetened condensed milk
equal volume of water
4 tsp citric acid (more or less to thicken)
1 tsp sea salt or to taste

Combine all ingredients in a glass screwtop jar and shake well to mix. Store in refrigerator. You can use malt vinegar instead of water with citric acid if you don't react to amines.

Basic white sauce

2 tbsp failsafe butter or margarine
1¹/₂ tbsp flour or gluten-free flour
1 cup or more of milk or milk substitute
sea salt to taste

Put butter in pan and stir until melted, add the flour to the butter, stir until cooked. The flour and butter have to be well cooked before adding liquid. Add liquid and whisk continually until thickened. Then add salt and remove from heat.

GRAVY AND TOMATO SAUCE SUBSTITUTES
Commercial gravies are very high in salicylates and amines and usually contain added MSG. Even home–made gravies are unsuitable because meat juices are high in amines. Use baby pear puree, or alternatives below.

Leek sauce

1 large leek, finely sliced
water
1 tsp butter
1 quantity of white sauce (above)

Cover microwave dish with leek slices. Add water until leek slices are just covered. Add butter. Microwave on high for 3 minutes. Make a white sauce and add leek mixture, stir well.

Birgit's pear chutney

Use instead of tomato sauce with sausages, other grilled meats and roast chicken.

1 large tin (825 g) of pears
   and syrup
$1/2$ cup brown sugar
2 tsp citric acid
1 tsp salt

Drain and dice pears. Put syrup in a saucepan and simmer until reduced by half. Add pears and remaining ingredients. Simmer about 15 minutes or until mixture thickens. Allow to cool. Store and use from freezer.

Variation: Pear ketchup: puree mixture in blender • Add chopped leeks, shallots and garlic to diced pears • for a thicker sauce, thicken with cornflour, gluten-free if necessary.

Citric lemon juice

Real lemon juice contains salicylates and amines. Bottled lemon juice as used in processed foods contains sulphites as well. Use this substitute in any recipe which calls for lemon juice.

4 tbsp warm water
1 tsp sugar
$3/4$ tsp citric acid or to taste
$1/4$ tsp ascorbic acid (vitamin C)
   powder, optional

Put sugar in warm water, stir to dissolve. Add remaining ingredients and store in refrigerator.

Quick chicken stock

Commercial chicken stock will always contain MSG, even if added as HVP and not listed. After a roast chicken, you can put the bones and neck in a saucepan with water and simmer for one hour. To reduce amine build up, cook no longer than necessary. Strain, cool and store in refrigerator or freezer, skim off fat.

Some Australian–American terms

FRUIT AND VEGETABLES

Choko: chayote, vegetable pear
Marrow: squash
Pawpaw: papaya
Rockmelon: cantaloupe
Shallots: green onions
Sultanas: golden raisins
Swedes: rutabaga

MISCELLANEOUS

Biscuits: crackers or cookies
Cordial: a drink base similar to Kool-Aid but sold as a liquid
Cornflour: corn starch
Cold pressed: expeller pressed
Fairy floss: cotton candy
Grilled: broiled
Icypoles: popsicles
Icing sugar: confectionery sugar
Icing: frosting
Lamingtons: cubes of sponge cake, normally covered in chocolate and coconut
Lamington tin, baking tray, swiss roll tin: similar in size to the American standard 13″ × 9″ pan
Muesli: granola
Paracetamol (Panadol): acetaminophen (Tylenol)
Rice Bubbles: Rice Krispies
Rissoles: beef or lamb pattie
Sports drinks: thirst quenchers
Soft drinks: sodas

Soda water: club soda
Scones: biscuits
Sweets, lollies, confectionery: candies

Nuttelex is a dairy free margarine made from safflower, sunflower and cottonseed oils, water, salt, emsulifiers 322, 471, flavour (vegetable), vitamins A and D, no added colour. It is very well tolerated by most food sensitive people. While in the US I found a similar product, if you can tolerate soy. Shedd's Willow Run dairy-free soybean margarine contains liquid soybean oil and partially hydrogenated soybean oil, water, salt, soybean flour, lecithin, betacarotene, vitamin A. For distributors, phone toll free 1800 735 3554.

Golden syrup is not available in the USA. Use rice malt or maple syrup.

Some failsafe food in the USA not available in Australia: natural maple candy; Wild Oats natural vanilla crème sandwich cookies (www.wildoats.com); many brands of uncoloured vanilla icecreams

Warning: Since September 2001, residents in the US have been warned to eat only very well cooked eggs because of the risk of Salmonella due to overcrowding. This means no more licking the bowl while making a cake, no soft-boiled eggs, eggs fried sunny-side up, softly scrambled or in omelettes and French toast. Avoid home-made mayonnaise and icecream with eggs. Some of the recipes in this chapter are not suitable for US eggs.

23 Food additives by code number

- **Bold** indicates additives which are most likely to cause adverse reactions. Avoid.
- *Italic* indicates new, untested additives. Avoid during your elimination diet and approach with caution.

Other additives are unlikely to cause reactions unless noted. There is a list of additives by name on www.fedupwithfood additives.info.

COLOURS

100   Turmeric or curcumin, yellow
101   Riboflavin, lactoflavin, Vitamin B2, yellow (failsafe)
102   Tartrazine, yellow #5 (AVOID)
103   Alkanet or alkannin pink

Alkanet is so new it hasn't been tested for behavioural and learning toxicity. It is a natural colour derived from a plant. As with annatto, this is no guarantee of safety.

104   Quinoline yellow (AVOID)
110   Sunset yellow (AVOID)
120   Cochineal or carmines, red

Cochineal, from the body of a South American insect, is moderate in terms of food intolerance reactions, but severe allergic reactions have been reported, especially in dye workers.

122   **Azorubine (AVOID)**
123   **Amaranth (AVOID)**
124   **Ponceau 4R (AVOID)**
127   **Erythrosine (AVOID)**
129   **Allura red (AVOID)**
132   **Indigotine (AVOID)**
133   **Brilliant blue (AVOID)**
140   Chlorophyll
141   Chlorophyll-copper
142   **Food green (AVOID)**
143   **Fast green**
150   *Caramel (see box below)*

Caramel 150 may be divided into 150a (plain or spirit caramel), 150b (caustic sulphite caramel) 150c (ammonia caramel) and 150d (ammonia sulphite caramel). Plain caramel is considered failsafe. There is a report of sulphite ammonia caramel used widely in soft drinks like cola causing problems for the extra sulphite sensitive.

---

151   **Brilliant black BN (AVOID)**
153   Carbon black, vegetable carbon (carbon withdrawn in the USA for possible cancer risk)
155   **Brown HT (AVOID)**
160a   Beta-carotene (failsafe)
160b   **Annatto extracts (AVOID)**
160c   *Paprika oleoresins (new)*
160d   *Lycopene (new)*
160e   *Beta-apo-8' carotenal (new)*
160f   *E-apo-8' carotenoic acid (new)*

160c, d, e, f are too new to have been tested for behavioural toxicity. They might be safe like beta-carotene (160a) or potentially harmful like annatto (160b).

161a   *Flavoxanthin, yellow (see comment)*
161b   *Lutein (new)*

161c   Kryptoxanthin (new)
161d   Rubixanthin (new)
161e   Violoxanthin (new)
161f   Rhodoxanthin (new)

Beta-apo-8'carotenal (160e) and xanthophylls not yet permitted in Australia, canthaxanthin (161g) and citranaxanthin (161i), are used in poultry feed to deepen the colour of egg yolks. I have received a few reports of reactions. Canthaxanthin taken in large quantities in tanning tablets has been associated with retinal damage. It is used as a food colour, in poultry feed and fed to farmed salmon and trout to colour their flesh. See sample colours in eggs at http://www.iceland.co.uk/Ext_11/web/Market.nsf/(WebSearch)/CusEggs/.

162   Beet red

Beet red may contain sodium nitrate (preservative 251) up to 25 mg/kg.

163   Anthocyanins, red, blue, violet (from plants)
164   Saffron, crocetin or crocin (failsafe)

Colours made from plants are moderate in salicylates (e.g. anthocyanins, beet red, turmeric, tannins) except for beta-carotene (160a) and saffron (164) which are low.

170   Calcium carbonate, white (failsafe)
171   Titanium dioxide, white (failsafe)
172   Iron oxide (black, red, yellow) (failsafe)
173   Aluminium
174   Silver
175   Gold
181   Tannic acid, brown

PRESERVATIVES—SORBATES
200   Sorbic acid (AVOID)
201   Sodium sorbate (AVOID)
202   Potassium sorbate (AVOID)
203   Calcium sorbate (AVOID)

PRESERVATIVES—BENZOATES
210   Benzoic acid (AVOID)
211   Sodium benzoate (AVOID)
212   Potassium benzoate (AVOID)
213   Calcium benzoate (AVOID)

Sorbates and benzoates have been associated with the full range of food intolerance reactions.

216   Propylparaben
218   Methylparaben

Preservatives 216 and 218 are only permitted in food colours in Australia.

PRESERVATIVES—SULPHITES
220   Sulphur dioxide (AVOID)
221   Sodium sulphite (AVOID)
222   Sodium bisulphite (AVOID)
223   Sodium metabisulphite (AVOID)
224   Potassium metabisulphite (AVOID)
225   Potassium sulphite (AVOID)
228   Potassium bisulphite (AVOID)

Sulphites (above) are the biggies for asthmatics. Not to be confused with sulphates (514–519).

234   Nisin
235   Natamycin or pimaricin
242   *Dimethyl dicarbonate (new, untested)*

PRESERVATIVES—NITRATES AND NITRITES (also colour fixatives)

249   Potassium nitrite (AVOID)
250   Sodium nitrite (AVOID)
251   Sodium nitrate (AVOID)
252   Potassium nitrate (AVOID)

Nitrates and nitrites are used in processed meats.

FOOD ACIDS

260   Acetic acid
261   Potassium acetate
262   Sodium acetates
263   Calcium acetate
264   Ammonium acetate
270   Lactic acid

PRESERVATIVES—PROPIONATES

280   Propionic acid (AVOID)
281   Sodium propionate (AVOID)
282   Calcium propionate (AVOID)
283   Potassium propionate (AVOID)

Widespread use in bread in Australia and the US, propionates are rarely used in Europe. Recently permitted also in cheese, fruit and vegetable products in Australia.

290   Carbon dioxide (propellant)
296   Malic acid (food acid)
297   Fumaric acid (food acid)

ANTIOXIDANTS

300   Ascorbic acid (Vitamin C)
301   Sodium ascorbate
302   Calcium ascorbate
303   Potassium ascorbate
304   Ascorbyl palmitate

306	Mixed tocopherols (Vitamin E)
307	Alpha tocopherol
308	Delta tocopherol
309	Gamma tocopherol
310	**Propyl gallate (AVOID)**
311	**Octyl gallate (AVOID)**
312	**Dodecyl gallate (AVOID)**
315	Erythorbic acid
316	Sodium erythorbate
319	**tert-Butylhydroquinone, TBHQ (AVOID)**
320	**Butylated hydroxyanisole, BHA (AVOID)**
321	**Butylated hydroxytoluene, BHT (AVOID)**
322	Lecithin (also an emulsifier)

Gallates and TBHQ, BHA and BHT are used to preserve vegetable oils and margarines. When vegetable oils are used in other products, these antioxidants are often unlisted because of the 5 per cent labelling loophole. BHA and BHT can also leach into products from cereal wrappers and clingfilm. Antioxidants 300–309 are safe alternatives.

MORE FOOD ACIDS

325	Sodium lactate
326	Potassium lactate
327	Calcium lactate
328	Ammonium lactate
329	Magnesium lactate
330	Citric acid
331	Sodium citrates
332	Potassium citrates
333	Calcium citrate
334	Tartaric acid
335	Sodium tartrate
336	Potassium tartrates
337	Potassium sodium tartrate
338	Phosphoric acid

Food acids are safe for most people. Most failsafers can manage citric acid (330), a few react.

MINERAL SALTS
339   Sodium phosphates
340   Potassium phosphates
341   Calcium phosphates
342   Ammonium phosphates
343   Magnesium phosphates

MORE FOOD ACIDS
349   Ammonium malate
350   Sodium malates
351   Potassium malate
352   Calcium malate
353   Metatartaric acid
354   Calcium tartrate
355   Adipic acid
357   Potassium adipate
359   Ammonium adipates
363   Succinic acid
365   Sodium fumarate
366   Potassium fumarate
367   Calcium fumarate
368   Ammonium fumarate
375   Nicotinic acid, niacin (B vitamin)
380   Ammonium citrates
381   Ferric ammonium citrate

ANOTHER PRESERVATIVE
385   Calcium disodium EDTA chelating agent, newly permitted in Australia

VEGETABLE GUMS AND THICKENERS
400   Alginic acid
401   Sodium alginate
402   Potassium alginate
403   Ammonium alginate
404   Calcium alginate
405   Propylene glycol alginate
406   Agar
407   Carrageenan
407a   Processed eucheuma seaweed
409   Arabinogalactan
410   Locust bean gum
412   Guar gum

Vegetable gums are failsafe. Guar and xanthan are used extensively by coeliacs. Carrageenan (407) used in yoghurts, ice-creams and others has been linked to cancer and is not recommended in large quantities for young children.

413   Tragacanth gum
414   Gum arabic (Acacia)
415   Xanthan gum
416   Karaya gum
418   Gellan gum

HUMECTANTS
420   Sorbitol
421   Mannitol
422   Glycerin (glycerol)

Humectants keep food moist. These additives are also used as sweeteners. The first two are not permitted in foods for babies and young children. Glycerin is used as a humectant in marshmallows and other sweets. All can cause nausea, bloating or severe diarrhoea, even when in chewing gum.

EMULSIFIERS
431   Polyoxyethylene (40) stearate
433   Polyoxyethylene (20) sorbitan monooleate
435   Polyoxyethylene (20) sorbitan monostearate
436   Polyoxyethylene (20) sorbitan tristearate
440   Pectin (also a vegetable gum)
442   Ammonium salts of phosphatidic acid
444   Sucrose acetate isobutyrate
445   Glycerol esters of wood rosins

MORE MINERAL SALTS
450   Pyrophosphates
451   Triphosphates
452   Polyphosphates
460   Cellulose microcrystalline and powdered (anti-caking agent)

THICKENERS, VEGETABLE GUMS

461   Methylcellulose
464   Hydroxypropyl methylcellulose
465   Methyl ethylcellulose
466   Sodium carboxymethylcellulose

EMULSIFIERS

470   Aluminium, calcium, sodium, magnesium, potassium and
      ammonium salts of fatty acids
471   Mono- and di-glycerides of fatty acids
472a Acetic and fatty acid esters of glycerol
472b Lactic and fatty acid esters of glycerol
472c Citric and fatty acid esters of glycerol
472e Diacetyltartaric and fatty acid esters of glycerol
472f Tartaric, acetic and fatty acid esters of glycerol (mixed)
473   Sucrose esters of fatty acids
475   Polyglycerol esters of fatty acids
476   Polyglycerol esters of interesterified ricinoleic acid
477   Propylene glycol esters of fatty acids
480   Dioctyl sodium sulphosuccinate
481   Sodium lactylates
482   Calcium lactylates
491   Sorbitan monostearate
492   Sorbitan tristearate

MINERAL SALTS

500   Sodium carbonates
501   Potassium carbonates
503   Ammonium carbonates
504   Magnesium carbonate (anti-caking agent, mineral salt)
507   Hydrochloric acid (acidity regulator)
508   Potassium chloride
509   Calcium chloride
510   Ammonium chloride
511   Magnesium chloride
512   Stannous chloride (colour retention agent)
514   Sodium sulphate (mineral salt)
515   Potassium sulphate (mineral salt)
516   Calcium sulphate (flour treatment agent, mineral salt)
518   Magnesium sulphate (mineral salt)
519   Cupric sulphate (mineral salt)
526   Calcium hydroxide (mineral salt)
529   Calcium oxide (mineral salt)

535	Sodium ferrocyanide (anti-caking agent)
536	Potassium ferrocyanide (anti-caking agent)
541	Sodium aluminium phosphate, acidic (acidity regulator, emulsifier)
542	Bone phosphate (anti-caking agent)
551	Silicon dioxide (anti-caking agent)
552	Calcium silicate (anti-caking agent)
553	Magnesium silicates (talc) (anti-caking agent)
554	Sodium aluminosilicate (anti-caking agent)
556	Calcium aluminium silicate (anti-caking agent)
558	Bentonite (anti-caking agent)
559	Aluminium silicate (kaolin) (anti-caking agent)
560	Potassium silicate
570	Stearic acid (anti-caking agent)
575	Glucono delta-lactone (acidity regulator)
577	Potassium gluconate (stabiliser)
578	Calcium gluconate (acidity regulator)
579	Ferrous gluconate (colour retention agent)
580	Magnesium gluconate
586	*4-hexylresorcinol*

FLAVOUR ENHANCERS

620	**L-Glutamic acid (AVOID)**
621	**Monosodium L-glutamate (MSG) (AVOID)**
622	**Monopotassium L-glutamate (AVOID)**
623	**Calcium di-L-glutamate (AVOID)**
624	**Monoammonium L-glutamate (AVOID)**
625	**Magnesium di-L-glutamate (AVOID)**
627	***Disodium guanylate (ribonucleotides)* (AVOID)**
631	***Disodium inosinate* (AVOID)**
635	***Disodium 5'-ribonucleotides (ribonucleotides)* (AVOID)**

The adverse effects of MSG (621) are well documented. I have also received many reports of skin rashes associated with new additive 635 which is a combination of 627 and 631.

636	Maltol
637	Ethyl maltol
640	Glycine
641	L-Leucine

MISCELLANEOUS ADDITIVES

900a   Polydimethylsiloxane (emulsifier, antifoaming agent, anti-caking agent)
901   Beeswax, white and yellow (glazing agent)
903   Carnauba wax (glazing agent)
904   Shellac, bleached (glazing agent)
905b   Petrolatum (glazing agent)
914   Oxidised polyethylene (humectant)
920   L-Cysteine monohydrochloride (flour treatment agent)

Former food additives 925 (chlorine), 926 (chlorine dioxide) and 928 (benzoyl peroxide), used as flour treatment agents, are now classified as bleaching/processing agents. Therefore, although they leave residues in your food, they will not appear on the label.

941   Nitrogen (propellant)
942   Nitrous oxide (propellant)

ARTIFICIAL SWEETENERS

950   Acesulphame potassium (artificial sweetening substance)
951   Aspartame (artificial sweetening substance) (AVOID)

The safety of aspartame with regard to brain tumours is not proven. There are reports of addiction; not recommended. Sugar is a natural alternative. Artificial sweeteners in general are unnecessary, artificial and not recommended.

952   Cyclamate (artificial sweetening substance)
953   Isomalt (humectant)
954   Saccharin (artificial sweetening substance)
955   Sucralose (artificial sweetening substance)
956   Alitame (artificial sweetening substance)
957   Thaumatin (flavour enhancer, artificial sweetening substance)

965   Maltitol and maltitol syrup (humectant, stabiliser)
966   Lactitol (humectant)

967   Xylitol (humectant, stabiliser)
968   Erythritol
1001   Choline salts and esters (emulsifier)
1100   Amylases (flour treatment agent)
1101   Proteases (papain, bromelain, ficin) (flour treatment agent, stabiliser, flavour enhancer)
1102   Glucose oxidase (antioxidant)
1104   Lipases (flavour enhancer)
1105   Lysozyme (preservative)
1200   Polydextroses (humectant)
1201   Polyvinylpyrolidone (stabiliser, clarifying agent, dispersing agent)

THICKENERS, VEGETABLE GUMS
1400   Dextrins roasted starch
1401   Acid treated starch
1402   Alkaline treated starch
1403   Bleached starch
1404   Oxidised starch
1405   Enzyme-treated starches
1410   Monostarch phosphate
1412   Distarch phosphate
1413   Phosphated distarch phosphate
1414   Acetylated distarch phosphate
1420   Starch acetate (esterified with acetic anhydride)
1422   Acetylated distarch adipate
1440   Hydroxypropyl starch
1442   Hydroxypropyl distarch phosphate
1450   Starch sodium octenylsuccinate
1505   Triethyl citrate

1518   Triacetin (humectant)
1520   Propylene glycol (humectant)
1521   Polyethylene glycol 8000 (antifoaming agent)

24 Checklist of common mistakes

If the diet isn't working as well as you expected, you need to talk to someone experienced who will check every item for you. If your dietitian won't do it, you are welcome to email me with a list of everything you eat in a typical day (sdengate@ozemail.com.au), but read the list below first. It is common for me to pick up at least five mistakes—just one mistake is enough to spoil the diet.

Not only foods
Prescription or over-the-counter medications containing colours, flavours or preservatives can affect you. Coloured (even pale pink) toothpaste is not permitted.

Unlabelled or illegal additives
It is not enough to read labels. Ask about all unpackaged and restaurant foods. If you don't trust your butcher, avoid mince (possible sulphites) or make your own.

Natural colour annatto (160b)
This colour is now in many dairy foods such as yoghurt and icecream, as well as cheese slices, frozen ovenbake chips and a wide variety of other processed foods. In the US, it is in a brand of croissants. Since it usually causes a reaction the next day, people don't realise if affects them.

Antioxidants (310–312, 319–321)
Not always listed on the label, these are used to preserve fats and oils. They are likely to be in any product which contains fats or 'vegetable oil' or specific oils like canola or sunflower oil (300–309 are failsafe). Low-fat crackers such as water crackers and wheat crackers contain less oil and are therefore safer but no commercial product is completely safe. It depends on how

much you eat. If no improvement, **avoid any commercial product containing any kind of vegetable oil, vegetable shortening, vegetable fat, beef fat or tallow** unless you are absolutely certain they are OK. Nearly all oils in New Zealand contain these additives.

Hot chips and potato crisps

Commercial hot chips can contain sulphites and will always contain harmful antioxidants. Make your own. Some crisps are failsafe (Kettle brand and Colvan). Watch out for 160b in ovenbake chips.

Sulphites in gelatine

Gelatine contains sulphur dioxide. You can drive this preservative off by dissolving gelatine in boiling water. Extra sensitive people will need to avoid gelatine and glucose syrup.

Too many salicylates

If you come from a food intolerant family, you are very likely to react to salicylates. Ignore well-meaning relatives, doctors and even some dietitians who say 'but an apple (or a carrot) a day won't hurt you'. It will. Worrying about nutrition is counter-productive in the first three weeks. Your most urgent need is to get rid of the food chemicals and the cravings. Stick to the low salicylate list. You won't see a reaction to one apple or one carrot—or even a regular intake of high-salicylate items like avocadoes—but you won't get the improvement you want, either. Or you will see an improvement but after a while the effects will build up and you'll be back to where you started. If you are worried about nutrition, eat permitted vegetables and take **permitted supplements only** during the strict elimination diet (Macro M multivitamins, Caltrate calcium supplements, available from pharmacies or www.pharmacydirect.com.au). Pear juice is NOT failsafe because commercial pear juice contains the peel. Pears canned in juice instead of syrup, like those handy little containers for lunchboxes, are NOT permitted. Pears and equivalent products (fresh, tinned, pureed, jam and ketchup) are limited to two pears per day, less for some people. Pears must be peeled, ripe, soft and juicy. A few people are *extremely* sensitive to salicylates and cannot tolerate any pear products or lemon juice-flavoured products. Treats like Darrell Lea white jelly beans (four per day) and 7UP (150 ml/week) are limited but avoid them altogether if you are not improving. Very sensitive people might have trouble with shallots, leeks, golden syrup and brown sugar but not white sugar. Others can manage pears but an apple or carrot every second day (**after** the elimination diet) will be too much. Sometimes these same people appear to be sugar sensitive.

Flavours

Artificial and natural flavours (e.g. natural fruit flavours) and even natural vanilla can cause problems (e.g. in vanilla yoghurt, custard, vanilla soymilk, soy icecream, and flavours in caramels, toffees, lollies and biscuits). White marshmallows other than Pascall's (limit four per day) contain too much artificial flavour. If your child is not improving, **avoid all commercial products containing 'flavour'** or use them as a *very occasional* treat, not every day. Rice Bubble Treats (LCMs) are permitted but I do receive complaints. If your child is not improving or is getting worse, avoid them. Home cooking is safer but avoid vanilla.

Mint or herbal flavoured toothpaste

If you can't get Soul Pattinson's plain, use salt. (After the elimination diet, you might manage Colgate white regular, rinse well, no sucking on the toothbrush). Herbal toothpastes like fennel from health food stores are not failsafe. All herbs contain salicylates.

Peter's Lemonade Icypoles

The recipe has changed. Avoid.

Commercial cashew paste

Must be made from raw cashews. Lightly roasted is not good enough.

Ingredient changes in commercial products

Beware, manufacturers can change ingredients at any time. For example, a brand of soymilk which was previously failsafe now uses dried cane juice which contains salicylates. Some others have started using cold-pressed oil and for a while an entire range of soymilks was not failsafe because of a switch to sunflower oil which contained TBHQ (319), not listed on the label because of the 5 per cent labelling loophole. The only way to keep up with these changes is to be on the newsletter mailing list or check 'Product Updates' at www.fedupwithfoodadditives.info.

One thing at a time

Avoid unnecessary medications and unnecessary visits to GPs, specialists, naturopaths, optometrists and dentists while you are doing your elimination diet. Most medications from GPs and paediatricians can interfere with the diet, especially in coloured or flavoured syrup form. Likewise, remedies from naturopaths. If they say their herbal remedies and vitamins are free from salicylates, they have a different definition of salicylates. Echinacea is just one herbal remedy which has been associated with a wide range of reactions from asthma to behaviour. Some diagnostic eye drops cause reactions. The dentist will probably use the wrong kind of toothpaste (you can take your own). Plaque disclosing tablets contain artificial colours. Worm your kids before you start the diet. Do not try to combine a candida diet and failsafe. Your efforts are more likely to be successful if you get failsafe 100 per cent right.

Carob

Many children react to carob buttons which contain 'flavours'. You can buy unflavoured buttons in some health food stores. Some people react to carob powder which is more bitter, tastes faintly of cinnamon and can have black flecks in it.

Rotisseried chicken with seasoning or stuffing

It is NOT OK to eat the meat and avoid the seasoning.

Natural fruit flavours

In vitamins or children's syrup medications, such as para-cetamol and cold medications and chewable vitamin tablets.

Herbal remedies and supplements

For example, Echinacea—if they contain herbs, they contain salicylates. Avoid. Fish oil supplements contain amines. Avoid. Take only failsafe supplements.

Accidental or deliberate mistakes

For example, spreads, hot chips, takeaways. This diet will not work unless it is followed strictly. You can try hot chips, for example, as a challenge after you have sorted out the salicylates and amines.

'Mistakes' at school

Are you sure your child isn't sneaking food at school? One desperate family tried the diet unsuccessfully three times before they discovered their daughter had been eating food like coloured snakes at school nearly every day. Some children do better on home detention for three weeks while doing the diet, which is how superintendent Peter Bennett achieved success with juvenile offenders in the UK.

Wholegrain/wheat cereals, bran cereals, wholemeal bread

Some children react badly to these, possibly because of an intolerance to a certain chemical in wholegrain wheat which is not present in refined flour. Limit (e.g. two biscuits of cereal every second day) or if no improvement, avoid. If you are worried about fibre, try rolled oats and Country Life Rye bread or Brumby's Bavarian Rye.

Raw sugar, dark brown sugar

White, soft brown, icing and caster sugars are failsafe. Raw sugar and dark brown sugar coloured with molasses contain salicylates and molasses contains sulphites. Avoid commercial products which contain raw sugar or dried cane syrup (soymilk, cereals).

Cold-pressed or expeller-pressed oil

These contain salicylates. The only safe cold-pressed oil is soy. Watch for cold-pressed oil in soymilk.

Whey powder (natural calcium propionate)

Whey powder when fermented can contain natural calcium propionate. You can't tell from the label. Avoid whey powder in bread and croissants. Avoid also bread containing vinegar.

Too many amines

Eating meats of uncertain age can be a problem for the amine sensitive: 'Turns out, I've been giving my kids meats with lots of amines for the past two years, including the last two months, when I was trying to be failsafe. We bought meats the day they arrived at our store, right off the truck, but when I investigated, some of them came from 1,000 miles away, in cartons that were refrigerated, not frozen. You can't believe (well, actually, I suppose you could) how much better my kids are now that we buy all our meats from a local butcher, who guarantees no more than 36 hours between slaughter and sale.'

Fermented products

Fermentation produces amines. Failsafe lists show that fermented products like wine, beer, soy sauce, tempeh and miso are not permitted but be careful also of sauerkraut, strong yoghurt and yeast-free bread. Despite seemingly failsafe ingredients (e.g. flour, water, salt), yeast-free bread is made by a long rising process which encourages fermentation. Note that baker's yeast is failsafe, candida is not an issue for failsafers, and yeasted bread is safer than yeast-free bread.

Fetta cheese is not failsafe!

My apologies, this is a mistake in *Fed Up*.

For people in the US

Cornflour means corn starch—refined white starch from corn. This is failsafe. A flour from corn (cornmeal) which is yellow is not failsafe.

You may need to exclude more foods

People with severe symptoms of any kind (health, behaviour, learning) may have to avoid dairy foods and/or wheat or gluten. A relative with coeliac disease or irritable bowel is a warning sign. One mother had been doing the diet with what she considered success for two years but still received complaints from school. When her sister was diagnosed as a coeliac, she removed gluten from her son's diet and he became a completely different person. Some people also need to exclude foods like soy or eggs.

For people who are gluten-free

Malt contains gluten so beware of cereals and soymilks containing malt. Also watch for cornflour in commercial products: assume it is wheaten cornflour unless otherwise specified, in Pascall's white marshmallows, honeycomb confectionery, baking powder except Ward's. Even a toast crumb in Nuttelex can affect very sensitive gluten responders. When eating out avoid gravies, sauces and anything with thickener.

Extra sensitivity

Some extra sensitive people react to citric acid, cashews, potatoes, rice, gelatine—not common, but it happens. A few people react to Kettle chips but can manage Colvan chips. Sunflower oil is safer than canola for these people. Many people report that more than one cup of decaf coffee a day is too much. If you are not improving and don't know why, make sure you don't eat these foods every day.

Challenges

Challenges can be inconclusive if the dose isn't big enough. For salicylates, you should consume at least six serves every day for a week of recommended foods, e.g. 150 ml of apple juice, 1 cup strawberries and other high salicylate-only fruits, 1 packet of Lifesavers, etc. For amines, two to three large ripe bananas and 60–120 grams of dark chocolate plus other amine containing foods such as canned tuna, chocolate drinks.

Exposure to environmental chemicals

Avoid environmental chemicals such as paints, food dyes in playdough and preschool paints on skin, household cleaners, workplace chemicals, or perfumes, e.g. in cosmetics, soaps, shampoos, deodorants or washing powders. Avoid garden pesticides and weedkillers, pesticides on pets, or smells of new or newly cleaned soft furnishings and carpets, new mattresses, cars, formaldehydes in pet shops and shopping malls. Some people are more sensitive than others. Do not renovate your house, have your carpet cleaned, buy new furniture or a new car while doing this diet. People with chemical overexposure may be more sensitive to pesticides on vegetables than to salicylates, others are the opposite. (Organic vegies are higher in salicylates.)

Exposure to smells

As above, plus the smell of strong spicy foods, vinegars, lawn clippings and strong smelling plants—herb plants, strongly fragrant flowers, eucalypts, e.g. 'peppermint' gum, pine trees particularly if freshly cut as in Christmas trees or in wood burning stoves as logs or smoke.

Too much stress

For children, this can come from confrontational parenting or teaching styles. Once the diet has kicked in, watch the *1–2–3 Magic* video (available from www.amazon.com) or do the Triple P Parenting course (www.triplep.net) to encourage positivity in the family.

Consider also non-food factors

Like absent fathers, moving (not a good time to do the diet), a new baby, bullying, criticism, punishment or lack of friends. Children on the diet need love, praise, exercise and lots of time with parents.

This checklist is updated regularly on my website, www. fedupwithfoodadditives.info. It also has hints for those with extreme sensitivity to salicylates and amines.

Notes and references

Abstracts of many of the articles mentioned below can be found in the Medline medical database: www.pubmed.com

1 Asthma is increasing

p. 3 'Nearly half'—Haby MM and others, Asthma in preschool children, *Thorax* 2001 Aug;56(8):589–95.

p. 3 National Asthma Council, *Asthma Management Handbook*, www.nationalasthma.org.au.

p. 3 Second highest—Woolcock AJ, Learning from asthma deaths, *BMJ* 1997 May 17;314(7092):1427–8.

p. 4 Robertson CF and others, Prevalence of asthma in regional Victorian schoolchildren, *Med J Aust* 1992 Jun 15;156(12):831–3.

p. 4 Hijazi N and others, Diet and childhood asthma in a society in transition: a study in urban and rural Saudi Arabia, *Thorax* 2000 Sep;55(9):775–9, free online at www.thoraxjnl.com.

p. 5 'More than 50 per cent'—Allen D and others, Adverse reactions to foods, *Med J Aust* 1984;141(5):S37–42.

p. 5 'Nearly 70 per cent'—Towns SJ and Mellis CM, Role of acetyl salicylic acid and sodium metabisulfite in chronic childhood asthma, *Pediatrics* 1984 May;73(5):631–7.

p. 5 Danish hospital study—Hoj L and others, A double-blind controlled trial of elemental diet in severe, perennial asthma, *Allergy* 1981;36:257–62.

pp. 6–7 Bahceciler NN and others, Predictors for the severity of bronchial hyperreactivity in childhood asthma, *Am J Crit Care Med* 2001;164:1150–3.

p. 7 The RPAH study—Hodge L and others, Assessment of food chemical intolerance in adult asthmatic subjects, *Thorax* 1996;51:805–9.

pp. 8–9 Food allergy and intolerance table based on information in Clarke L and others, The dietary management of food allergy and food intolerance in children and adults, *Aust J Nutr Diet* 1996;53(3):89–94.

p. 11   Timberlake CM and others, Precipitation of asthma attacks in Melanesian adults by sodium metabisulphite, *P N G Med J* 1992 Sep;35(3):186–90.

p. 11   Steinman HA and others, Sulphur dioxide sensitivity in South African asthmatic children, *S Afr Med* J 1993 Jun;83(6):387–90.

2 The asthma additive

p. 13   ISAAC steering committee, Worldwide variation in prevalence of symptoms of asthma, allergic rhinoconjunctivitis and atopic eczema, *Lancet* 1998;351:1225–36.

p. 13   Beasley R and others, Prevalence and etiology of asthma, *J Allergy Clin Immunol* 2000;105:S466–72.

p. 14   Ellwood P and others, Diet and asthma, allergic rhinoconjunctivitis and atopic eczema symptom prevalence. *Eur Respir J* 2001;17:436–43.

p. 14   Stewart AW and others, The relationship of per capita gross national product to the prevalence of symptoms of asthma and other atopic diseases in children (ISAAC), *Int J Epidemiol* 2001;30: 173–9.

p. 15   Leclerq C and others, Dietary intake exposure to sulphites in Italy, *Food Addit Contam*, 2000;17(12):979–89.

p. 16   Ronchetti R and others, Is the increase in childhood asthma coming to an end? *Eur Respir J* 2001;17(5):881–6.

p. 16   A survey by the Australian Consumers Association in 1999 found nearly one third of sausages tested contained more than the legal limit of sulphite preservative. The test is from 1999 and the results were accurate at that time only. Reprinted from CHOICE Jan/Feb 1999 with the permission of the Australian Consumers' Association (ACA).

p. 16   Sulphites are illegal in fresh minced meat, but a 1994 survey found a maximum of 890 ppm, nearly twice what is allowed in sausages. Australia New Zealand Food Authority, *1994 Australian Market Basket Survey,* 1996, Australian Government Publishing Service, Canberra.

p. 16   Zubeldia Lauzurica L and others, Presence of sulfites in minced meat and meat products prepared in industries of the Valencia community, *Rev Espana Salud Publica* 1997;71(4):401–7 and Armentia-Alvarez A and others, Residual levels of free and total sulphite in fresh and cooked burgers. *Food Addit Contam* 1993;10(2):157–65.

p. 17   CSPI is a nonprofit consumer organisation based in Washington, D.C. focusing on food safety and nutrition: www.cspinet.org.

p. 17   Duke University research—Corder H and Buckley CE, Aspirin, Salicylate, sulfite and tartrazine induced bronchoconstriction, *J Clin Epidem* 1995;48(10):1269–75.

p. 18   Williams R, *Headaches, asthma, fries and a cola: the tale of the brimstone demons*, Rybett Controls, Inc. 2000. http://members.aol.com/nosulfites.

p. 18   Iyengar F and McEvily AJ, Anti-browning agents: alternative to the use of sulfites in foods.

p. 18   *Low sulphite Australian wines*: www.glenara.com.au.

3 Sulphites up close and personal

p. 21   Karen's story is from *Sulfites: Safe for Most, Dangerous for Some* by Ruth Papazian, FDA website: www.fda.gov.com.

p. 21   Melbourne survey—Woods RK and others, Patients' perceptions of food-induced asthma, *Aust NZ J Med* 1996;26:508–12.

p. 21   Duke University research—see Notes for Chapter 2.

p. 22   South African study—Steinman, see Notes for Chapter 1.

p. 23   Children's Hospital—Towns and Mellis, see Notes for Chapter 1.

p. 24   No sulfites—see Notes for Chapter 2.

p. 25   Swiss diet study—Genton G and others, Value of oral provocation tests to aspirin and food additives in the routine investigation of asthma and chronic urticaria, *J Allergy Clin Immunol* 1985;76(1):40–5.

4 Colour me asthmatic

p. 29   FDA approved petition to ban tartrazine by Ryan's mother, see p. 301.

p. 29   First reports in Dr S Speer's 1958 book, *Management of Childhood Asthma*, cited in Feingold B, Recognition of food additives as a cause of symptoms of allergy, *Ann Allergy* 1968;26:309–13; Yellow-coated vitamin tablet—Chafee FH and Settipane GA, Asthma caused by FD&C approved dyes. *J Allergy* 1967;40(2):65–72; Freedman BJ, Asthma induced by sulphur dioxide, benzoate and tartrazine contained in orange drinks. *Clin Allergy* 1977;7:407–15.

p. 29   Production of food colours, FDA figures quoted in Jacobson M and Schardt D, Diet, ADHD and Behaviour: a quarter-century review, *Centre for Science in the Public Interest*, 1999, www.cspinet.org.

p. 30   'misleading' FDA pamphlet on food colours—Jacobson MF and Schardt D, Diet, ADHD and behaviour: a quarter century review, 1999, Centre for Science in the Public Interest, Washington DC, piii (free download from www.cspinet.org).

p. 30   Ward NI and others, Assessment of chemical factors in relation to child hyperactivity, *J Nutr Envir Med* 1997;7(4):333–42.

p. 30   English curry houses—www.bbcnews.com.

p. 33   Mikkelsen H and others, Hypersensitivity reactions to food colours with special reference to the natural colour annatto extract (butter colour), *Arch Toxicol Suppl* 1978;(1):141–3.

p. 34   colour of eggs—see www.bbcnews.com and search for canthaxanthin, also http://www.iceland.co.uk/Ext_11/web/Market.nsf/(WebSearch)/CusEggs/.

p. 35   Up to 30 per cent react to tartrazine—Stenius S and Lemola M, Hypersensitivity to acetylsalicylic acid (ASA) and tartrazine in patients with asthma, *Clin Allergy* 1976;6(2):119–29.

p. 35   Realistic dose of food colours—Swanson J and Kinsbourne M, Food dyes impair performance of hyperactive children on a laboratory learning test, *Science* 1980;207:1485–7.

p. 35   Increase in food colours—according to FDA data, per capita production of food dyes has increased from 12 mg in 1955, to 32 mg in 1975, to 47 mg in 1998, a fourfold increase over four decades. Quoted in the CSPI report, above.

p. 36   Howard, Theresa, Kids salivate for new, yucky, weirdly coloured food, *USA Today*, 23/4/01, 7B.

5 More preservatives

p. 38   First mention of benzoate and asthma in Freedman, 1977, see Notes for Chapter 4.

p. 38   Petrus M and others, Asthme et intolérance aux benzoates, *Arch Pédiatr* 1996;3:984–7.

p. 39   Antioxidants and asthma—Fisherman EW and Cohen G, Chemical intolerance to butylated-hydroxyanisole (BHA) and butylated-hyroxytoluene (BHT) and vascular response as an indicator and monitor of drug intolerance, *Ann Allergy* 1973;31(3):126–33.

p. 40   Hawkins CA and Katelaris CH, Nitrate anaphylaxis, *Ann Allergy Asthma Immunol* 2000;85(1):74–6.

p. 40   Dengate S and Ruben A, Controlled trial of cumulative behavioural effects of a common bread preservative, *J Paediatr Child Health* 2002;38(4):373–6.

p. 42   PT's story—Baker GJ and others, Bronchospasm induced by metabisulphite-containing foods and drugs, *Med J Aust* 1981;2: 614–16.

6 Monosodium glutamate (MSG)

p. 45   Allen D, Delohery J and Baker G, Monosodium L-glutamate-induced asthma. *J Allergy Clin Immunol* 1987;80(4):530–7; the book by Schwartz GR, *In bad taste: The MSG Syndrome*, 1988, Signet, New York includes an account of this research by Dr Gary Baker.

p. 46   Increased forty-fold—www.NOMSG.com; world production of MSG is now estimated at nearly one million tons per year—Ninomiya K, An overview of recent research on MSG, *Food Aust* 2001;53(12):549.

p. 47   '. . . more than Japan or Korea' in Woods RK, MSG and asthma—what is the evidence? *Food Aust* 2001;53(12):555–9.

p. 47   Extreme users—Rhodes J and others, A survey of the monosodium glutamate content of foods and an estimation of the dietary intake of monosodium glutamate, *Food Addit Contam* 1991; 8(5):663–72.

p. 47   Everyone will react—Schaumburg HH and others, Monosodium l-Glutamate: its pharmacology and role in Chinese restaurant syndrome, *Science* 1969;163:826–8.

p. 48   25% react—Reif-Lehrer L, A questionnaire study of the prevalence of Chinese restaurant syndrome, *Fed Proc* 1977;36(5): 1617–23.

pp. 48–52   For the information in this chapter, I am much indebted to the hard work of Dr Samuels, published in Samuels A, The toxicity/safety of processed free glutamic acid (MSG): a study in suppression of information, *Accountability in Research* 1999;6: 259–310, free at www.truthinlabeling.org/l-manuscript.htm.

p. 48   The International Glutamate Technical Committee—see http://www.ajinomoto.co.jp/ajinomoto/A-Company/newman/ company/archv/usa.html and the Kellen company (association management) client list (www.kellencompany.com); activities listed in the Encyclopedia of Associations, quoted in Samuels, 1999, above for IGTC 1992; The Glutamate Association is described thus in The Google directory, www.google.com; www.truthinlabeling.org gives an alternative viewpoint to that of the International Glutamate Information Service, described in Samuels A, How safe is glutamate? *New Scientist*, 2002;176(2370):28; award-winning science website— http://biotch.icmb.utexas.edu/pages/scitools.html; 'particularly targeted'—Samuels, 1999, above; websites accessed November 2002.

p. 48   Less than 2% react—Kerr GR and others, Prevalence of the 'Chinese restaurant syndrome', *J Am Diet Assoc* 1979;75(1):29–33.

p. 50   'Consumer groups first heard' in Samuels, 1999, above.

p. 50   The study tested 100 asthmatics—Woessner KM, Simon RA and Stevenson DD, Monosodium glutamate sensitivity in asthma, *J Allergy Clin Immunol* 1999;104(2 Pt 1):305–10.

p. 50   Review . . . criticising . . .—Stevenson DD, Monosodium glutamate and asthma, *J Nutr* 2000;130:1067S–73S.

p. 51   Disclosure of company ties—Editorial, Sponsorship, authorship and accountability, *Lancet* 2001;358(9285):854; Relman A, Trust me, I'm a Scientist, *New Scientist*, 2001;171(2308):46–7.

p. 53   Box—Moneret-Vautrin DA, Monosodium glutamate-induced asthma, *Allerg Immunol* 1987;19(1):29–35, all others in Notes for this chapter except Hodge and others, see Notes for Chapter 1.

p. 53   Melbourne asthmatics' perceptions, see Woods, Notes for Chapter 2.

p. 53   Results resembled—Woods RK and others, The effects of monosodium glutamate in adults with asthma who perceive themselves to be monosodium glutamate-intolerant, *J Allergy Clin Immunol* 1998;101:762–71.

pp. 53–54   Woods RK, MSG and asthma—what is the evidence? *Food Aust* 2001;53(12):555–9, in The Future of MSG, 'publication sponsored by the International Glutamate Information Service', *Food Aust* 2001; 53(12);545–59.

7 Salicylates and amines

p. 57 Scripps clinic—McDonald JR, Mathison DA and Stevenson DD, Aspirin intolerance in asthma, *J Allergy Clin Immunol* 1972;50(4): 198–207.

p. 58 Sakakibara H, and Suetsugu S, Aspirin-induced asthma is an important type of bronchial asthma, *Nihon Kyobu Shikkan Gakkai Zasshi* 1995;33(Suppl:)106–15.

p. 59 Swain AR and others, Salicylates in foods, *J Am Diet Assoc* 1985;85:950–60.

p. 59 Feingold list incomplete—Gibson A and Clancy R, Management of chronic idiopathic urticaria by the identification and exclusion of dietary factors, *Clin Allergy* 1980;10:699–704.

p. 59 Peppermint and honey—Burr ML and others, Food-allergic asthma in general practice, *Hum Nutr Appl Nutr*, 1985; 39(5):349–55.

p. 59 Toothpaste sensitivity—Inagaki M and others, Inhibitory effect of amlexanox on asthmatic attacks in an aspirin sensitive asthmatic, *Nihon Kyobu Shikkan Gakkai Zasshi* 1992;30(6):1180–5. Abstract (article in Japanese).

p. 60 Chan TY, Potential dangers from topical preparations containing methyl salicylate, *Hum Exp Toxicol* 1996;15(9):747–50.

p. 60 Shelley WB, Birch pollen and aspirin psoriasis, *JAMA* 1964; 189(13):985–8.

p. 61 Zeitz HJ, Bronchial asthma, nasal polyps and aspirin sensitivity: Samter's syndrome, *Clin Chest Med* 1988;9(4):567–76.

p. 61 Samter M, Aspirin, salicylates and the magic of diets, *Cutis* 1977;20(1):18,24,52.

p. 61 Children's Hospital study, see Towns and Mellis, Notes for Chapter 1.

p. 65 Increasing salicylate levels in crops—Day S, Fight the Blight, *New Scientist* 2001;171(2306):36–9.

p. 66 Salicylates, amines and FI—Loblay RH and Swain AR, Food intolerance, *Recent Advances Clin Nutr* 1986;2:169–77.

8 Dairy foods

p. 68 Asthmatics say foods affect them, described in: Woods RK and others, Patients' perceptions of food-induced asthma, *Aust NZ J Med* 1996;26:504–12; Dawson KP, Childhood asthma: what do parents add or avoid in their children's diets? *NZ Med J* 1990;103:239–40.

p. 68 Asthmatic allergy to milk (one in 50)—Yazicioglu M and others, Egg and milk allergy in asthmatic children, *Allergol Immunopathol* (Madr) 1999 Nov–Dec;27(6):287–93; One in 38—May CD, Objective clinical and laboratory studies of immediate hypersensitivity reactions to foods in asthmatic children, *J Allergy Clin Immunol* 1976;58(4):500–15.

p. 69 Hill DJ and others. Manifestations of milk allergy in infancy: clinical and immunologic findings, *J Pediatr* 1986;109(2):270–6.

p. 71 Doctors say dairy foods affect asthmatics—combined National Asthma Council and Australian Dairy Corporation campaign, www.nac.com.au.

p. 71 Woods RK and others, Do dairy products induce bronchoconstriction in adults with asthma? *J Allergy Clin Immunol* 1998;101:45–50.

p. 73 'No medical foundation [for milk makes mucus]'—in the Diet and Asthma section of the NAC's Asthma Management Handbook, http://www.nationalasthma.org/publications/amh/st_det.htm.

p. 73 Pinnock CB and others, Relationship between milk intake and mucus production in adult volunteers challenged with rhinovirus-2, *Am Rev Respir Dis* 1990 Feb;141(2):352–6.

p. 74 Ear infections, in Washington—Nsouli TM and others, Role of food allergy in serous otitis media, *Ann Allergy* 1994 Sep;73(3):215–9; in Finland—Juntti H and others, Cow's milk allergy is associated with recurrent otitis media during childhood, *Acta Otolaryngol* 1999;119(8):867–73.

p. 74 Del Mar C and Glasziou P, A child with earache, *Aust Fam Phys* 2002;31(2):141–4.

p. 75 CSPI review—Leibman B, Bare bones: how to keep yours strong, *Nutrition Action* 2002;20(1):1–8.

p. 75 Rosemary Stanton's comments about soymilk in *Australian Doctor* reported in *Pritikin Lifestyle*, May 99, p. 6.

p. 76 Asthma medications and bone loss—Israel E and others,

Effects of inhaled glucocorticoids on bone density in premenopausal women, *N Engl J Med* 2001;345(13):941–7.

p. 77   Professor Fiatarone . . . considers—in Callaghan G, Close to the Bone, *Weekend Australian Magazine*, 6–7/7/02, pp. 32–35.

p. 77   Sellmeyer D and others, A high ratio of dietary animal to vegetable protein increases the rate of bone loss and the risk of fracture in postmenopausal women, *Am J Clin Nutr* 2001;73:118–22.

p. 78   Fox D, Hard cheese, *New Scientist*, 2001;172(2321):42–5.

9 Medication can be a health hazard

p. 80   Third leading cause of death—Starfield B, Is US health really the best in the world? *JAMA* 2000;284(4):483–4.

p. 80   Medication side effects—Lazarou J and others, Adverse drug reactions in hospitalised patients, *JAMA* 1998;270(15): 1200–5.

p. 80   Siegel-Itzkovich J. Doctors' strike in Israel may be good for health. *BMJ* 2000;320:1561, similarly in Canada, the US and South America. Full text at http://bmj.com/cgi/content/full/320/7249/1561.

p. 80   Safety of new drugs not guaranteed—Lasser, 2002, see box p. 80.

p. 80   Gifts–Wazana, 2000, see box p. 00.

p. 80   Side effects, rules of drug taking—Public Citizen www.citizen.org/hrg.

p. 82   Trautlein JJ, Mann WJ, Anaphylactic shock caused by yellow dye in an enema, *Ann Allergy* 1978 Jul;41(1):28–9.

p. 82   Ribon A and Parikh S, Drug-induced asthma: a review, *Ann Allergy* 1980;44:220–4.

p. 83   Hanssen M, *New Additive Code Breaker*, Lothian, 1991.

p. 83   Erythrosine—Weber RW and others, Incidence of bronchoconstriction due to aspirin, azo dyes, non-azo dyes, and preservatives in a population of perennial asthmatics, *J Allergy Clin Immunol* 1979;64(1):32–7.

p. 84   Antibiotics for earache—Del Mar, see Notes for Chapter 8.

p. 84   Schwartz HJ and others, Metabisulfite sensitivity and local dental anesthesia, *Ann Allergy*, 1989;62(2):83–6.

p. 85   Salicylates in drugs, see Ribon and Parikh above.

p. 86   Safety of paracetamol—Moynihan R, FDA fails to reduce accessibility of paracetamol despite 450 deaths a year, BMJ 2002;325(7366):678, free at http://bmj.com/cgi/content/full/325/7366/678.

pp. 88–89   Carson HJ and others, Death from asthma associated with sertraline overdose, *Am J Forensic Med Pathol* 2000;21(3):273–5.

p. 89   Katayuma H and others, Near death asthmatic reaction induced by disodium cromoglycate, *Intern Med* 1996;35(12):976–8.

p. 89   Hammer HB and others, Churg-Strauss syndrome after treatment with Singulair (montelukast), *Tidsskr Nor Laegeforen* 2002;122(5):484–6.

p. 90   Sulfite-containing drugs in the US—American Academy of Pediatrics, see box, p. 90.

p. 91   Beasley R and others, Preservatives in nebulizer solutions: risks without benefit, *Pharmacotherapy,* 1998;18(1):130–9.

p. 91   Dickinson BD and others, Safety of over-the-counter inhalers for asthma, *Chest* 2000;118:522–6.

p. 91   Steroids—Schonwald S, Methylprednisolone anaphylaxis, *Am J Emerg Med* 1999;17(6):583–5.

p. 92   Hospital food—Hoj, see Notes for Chapter 1.

10 A call to arms

p. 94   Survey in 1997, reported in—Downs SH and others, Continued increase in the prevalence of asthma and atopy, *Arch Dis Child* 2001;84:20–3.

p. 94   National Asthma Campaign, Report on the cost of asthma in Australia, NAC 1992.

p. 94   Half of asthmatic adults (Hoj, Allen), two-thirds of children (Towns and Mellis), see Notes for Chapter 1.

p. 95   Farrer KTH, Food additives debate in Victoria 100 years ago, *Food Aust* 2001;53(6):217–19.

p. 96   Safe and effective alternatives to artificial colours—Evans K, New developments in natural colours for confectionery, *Food Aust* 1998;50(4):174.

p. 96   Alternatives to sulphites in all foods except wine, Leclerq, see Notes for Chapter 2.

p. 96   'Experiment in prevention—Beasley R and others, Withdrawal of fenoterol and the end of the New Zealand asthma mortality epidemic, *Int Arch Allergy Immunol* 1995 May–Jun;107(1–3):325–7.

11 Asthma can be fatal

p. 101   Bucknall CE and others, Scottish confidential inquiry into asthma deaths, *Thorax* 1999;54:978–84.

p. 101   Severity—National Asthma Campaign, *Report on the cost of asthma in Australia*, NAC, 1992.

pp. 101–15   Information on drugs and devices—www.nationalasthma.org.au, asthma foundation handouts, www.mydr.com.au and medical journals.

p. 104   Kamps AW and others, Peak flow diaries in childhood asthma are unreliable, *Thorax* 2001;56(3):180–2.

p. 105   Hancox RJ and others, Bronchodilator tolerance and rebound bronchoconstriction during regular inhaled beta-agonist treatment, *Respir Med* 2000;94(8):767–71.

p. 106   Beasley R and others, Beta agonists: what is the evidence that their use increases the risk of asthma morbidity and mortality? *J Allergy Clin Immunol* 1999;104(2 part 2):S18–S30.

p. 107   Side effects of Corticosteroids—www.nationaljewish.org/medfacts/corticosteroids.html; www.dermnetz.org/dna.systemic.steroids/ssteroids.html; Kayani S and Shannon DC, Adverse behavioural effects of treatment for acute exacerbation of asthma in children, *Chest*, 2002;122(2):624–8.

p. 108   Reinus JF and others, Severe liver injury after treatment with the leukotriene receptor antagonist zafirlukast, *Ann Intern Med* 2000;133(12):964–8.

p. 109   Churg-Strauss Syndrome, see Hammer, Notes for Chapter 9.

p. 113   Woolcock AJ and others, The burden of asthma in Australia, *Med J Aust*, 2001;175:141–5, available free at www.mja.com.au.

12 Asthma in babies and children

p. 117   Bjorksten B and others, The intestinal microflora in allergic Estonian and Swedish 2-year-old children, *Clin Exp Allergy* 1999 Mar;29(3):342–6.

p. 117   Gewolb IH and others, Stool microflora in extremely low birth-weight infants, *Arch Dis Child Fetal Neonatal Ed* 1999;80(3):F167–73.

p. 117   Oddy WH and others, Maternal asthma, infant feeding, and the risk of asthma in childhood, *J Allergy Clin Immunol* 2002;110(1):65–7; a report at http://www.breastfeeding.asn.au/bfinfo/asthma.html.

p. 117   Sears MR and others, Long-term relation between breast-feeding and development of atopy and asthma in children and young adults, *Lancet* 2002;360(9337):901–7.

p. 118   Kleessen B and others, Influence of two infant formulas and human milk on the development of the faecal flora in newborn infants, *Acta Paediatr* 1995;84(12):1347–56.

p. 118   Chandra RK, Five-year follow-up of high-risk infants with family history of allergy who were exclusively breast-fed or fed partial whey hydrolysate, soy, and conventional cow's milk formulas, *J Pediatr Gastroenterol Nutr* 1997 Apr;24(4):380–8.

p. 118   Melsom T and others, Asthma and indoor environment in Nepal, *Thorax* 2001 Jun;56(6):477–81.

p. 118   Riedler J and others, Exposure to farming in early life and development of asthma and allergy, *Lancet 2001* Oct 6;358(9288): 1129–33.

p. 119   Droste JH and others, Does the use of antibiotics in early childhood increase the risk of asthma and allergic disease? *Clin Exp Allergy* 2000 Nov;30(11):1547–53.

p. 119   McKeever TM and others, The importance of prenatal exposures on the development of allergic disease, *Am J Respir Crit Care Med* 2002;166(6):827–32.

p. 119   Antibiotics for ear infections, Del Mar, see Notes for Chapter 8.

p. 119   Kalliomaki M and others, Probiotics in primary prevention of atopic disease, *Lancet* 2001 Apr 7;357(9262):1057–9.

p. 120   Hatakka K, Effect of long term consumption of probiotic milk on infections in children attending day care centres, *BMJ* 2001 Jun 2;322(7298):1327.

p. 121   Vanderhoof JA and others, Lactobacillus GG in the prevention of antibiotic-associated diarrhoea in children, *J Pediatr* 1999 Nov;135(5):564–8.

p. 122   Mellis CM, Is asthma prevention possible with dietary manipulation? *Med J Aust* 2002;177(6 Suppl):S78–80, available free through www.pubmed.com.

p. 122   Hodge L and others, Consumption of oily fish and childhood asthma risk, *Med J Aust* 1996;164:137–40.

p. 122   Takemura Y and others, The relationship between fish intake and the prevalence of asthma, *Prev Med* 2002 Feb;34(2):221–5.

p. 122   Nagakura T and others, Dietary supplementation with fish oil rich in omega-3 polyunsaturated fatty acids in children with bronchial asthma, *Eur Respir* 2000;16(5):861–5.

13 Asthma in adults

p. 125   Asthma in adults, Woolcock, see Notes for Chapter 11.

p. 125   Troisi RJ and others, Menopause, postmenopausal estrogen preparations, and the risk of adult-onset asthma, *Am J Respir Crit Care Med* 1995;152(4 Part 1):1183–8.

pp. 126–28   Field GB, Occupational Asthma, *Med J Aust*, 1984;141 (5 Suppl):S42–4.

p. 127   Banks DE and Wang ML, Occupational asthma: 'the big picture', *Occup Med* 2000;15(2):335–58.

p. 127   Miller ME and others, Occupational asthma caused by FD&C blue dye no. 2, *Allergy Asthma Proc* 1996;17(1):31–4.

p. 128   Alonso E and others, Baker's asthma in a child. *Allergol Immunopathol (Madr)* 2001;29(4):141–3.

p. 129   Senthilselvan A, Association of asthma with use of pesticides, *Am Rev Respir Dis* 1992;146(4):884–7.

p. 129   Bryant DH, Asthma due to insecticide sensitivity, *Aust NZ J Med* 1985;15:66–8.

p. 129   Karjalainen A and others, Work is related to a substantial portion of adult-onset asthma incidence in the Finnish population, *Am J Respir Crit Care Med* 2001;164(4):565–8.

14 Asthma in Australian Aborigines

p. 132   Valery P and others, Asthma is not prevalent in Aboriginal and Torres Strait Islander children: a myth, *J Paediatr Child Health* 2002; 38(1):105–6.

p. 132   Downs SH and others, Asthma and hayfever in Aboriginal and non-Aboriginal children living in non-remote rural towns, *Med J Aust* 2001;175(1):10–13.

p. 132   Valery P and others, High prevalence of asthma in five remote Indigenous communities in Australia, *Eur Resp J* 2001;17:1–9.

p. 132   Veale AJ and others, Asthma and atopy in four rural Australian Aboriginal communities, *Med J Aust* 1996;165:192–6.

p. 132   Gracey M, A pediatrician and his mothers and his infants, *Turk J Pediatr* 1997;39(1):1–5.

pp. 132–34   Shortwind project, see website www.asthmant.org.au or contact Asthma NT, p. 299.

15 Worst case scenario: anaphylaxis

p. 137   Brazil E and MacNamara AF, 'Not so immediate' hypersensitivity—the danger of biphasic anaphylactic reactions, *J Accid Emerg Med* 1998;15:252–3.

p. 137   Brown AF and others, Emergency department anaphylaxis, *Allergy Clin Immunol* 2001 Nov;108(5):861–6.

p. 138   Sampson HA, Food anaphylaxis, *Br Med Bull* 2000;56(4): 925–35.

p. 138   Kemp SF and others, Anaphylaxis. A review of 266 cases, *Arch Intern Med* 1995;155(16):1749–54.

pp. 138–39   Laoprasert N and others, Anaphylaxis in a milk-allergic child following ingestion of lemon sorbet containing trace quantities of milk, *J Food Prot* 1998;61(11):1522–4.

p. 139   Jarmoc LM and Primack WA, Anaphylaxis to cutaneous exposure to milk protein in a diaper rash ointment, *Clin Pediatr (Phila)* 1987 Mar;26(3):154–5.

p. 139   Kemp AS and others, Anaphylaxis caused by inhaled pavlova mix in egg-sensitive children, *Med J Aust* 1988;149(11–12):712–3.

p. 139   Hidden peanuts—Wuthrich B and Ballmer-Weber BK, Food-induced anaphylaxis, *Allergy* 2001;56(Suppl 67):102–4.

p. 139   Desmond RE and Trautlein JJ, Tartrazine (FD&C yellow #5) anaphylaxis, *Ann Allergy* 1981;46:81–2.

p. 139   Bennett AT and Collins KA, An unusual case of anaphylaxis. Mold in pancake mix, *Am J Forensic Med Pathol* 2001;22(3): 292–5.

p. 140   Drain KL and Volcheck GW, Preventing and managing drug-induced anaphylaxis, *Drug Saf* 2001;24(11):843–53.

p. 140   Van Puijenbroek EP and others, Different risks for NSAID-induced anaphylaxis, *Ann Pharmacother* 2002;36(1):24–9, Netherlands Pharmacovigilance Foundation.

p. 141   Levy MB and Fink JN, Anaphylaxis to celecoxib, *Ann Allergy Asthma Immunol* 2001;87(1):72–3.

p. 141   Ford SA and others, Anaphylactic or anaphylactoid reactions in patients undergoing cardiac surgery, *J Cardiothorac Vasc Anesth* 2001;15(6):684–8.

p. 141   Sakaguchi M and Inouye S, Anaphylaxis to gelatin-containing rectal suppositories, *J Allergy Clin Immunol* 2001;108(6):1033–4.

p. 141   Cimmino VM and others, Allergic reactions to isosulfan blue during sentinel node biopsy—a common event, *Surgery* 2001; 130(3):439–42.

p. 141   Smolinske SC, Review of parenteral sulfite reactions, J *Toxicol Clin Toxicol* 1992;30(4):597–606. Micromedex, POISINDEX Information System, Denver, CO.

p. 142   Fiocchi A and others, Severe anaphylaxis induced by latex as a contaminant of plastic balls in play pits, *J Allergy Clin Immunol* 2001;108(2):298–300.

p. 142   Konrad C and others, Latex allergy—not only a threatening danger to patients, *Schweiz Rundsch Med Prax* 1996;85(15):482–5.

p. 142   Free S, Latex allergy: what it could mean for you, *Aust Crit Care* 1998;11(2):40–3.

p. 144   Hawkins CA and Katelaris CH, Nitrate anaphylaxis, *Ann Allergy Asthma Immunol* 2000;85(1):74–6.

p. 145   Peanut allergy, from Figleaf (Food Intolerance Group) newsletter.

p. 146   English survey—Pumphrey RS, Lessons for management of anaphylaxis from a study of fatal reactions, *Clin Exp Allergy* 2000;30(8):1144–50.

16 Breathing lessons

p. 148   Moynihan, R. 'Drug seller defection', *Australian Financial Review*, 23/8/01, p. 61; http://www.asthmacare.ie/detailedPress Releases.htm#11.

p. 149   Van Dixhoorn J and Duivenvoorden HJ, Efficacy of the Nijmegen questionnaire in recognition of the hyperventilation syndrome, *Psychosomatic Res* 1985;29:199–206.

p. 149   Thomas M and others, Prevalence of dysfunctional breathing in patients treated for asthma in primary care, *BMJ* 2001;322: 1098–100.

p. 149   Manocha M and others, Sahaja yoga in the management of moderate to severe asthma, *Thorax* 2002;57(2):110–15.

p. 149   Mater study—Bowler SD and others, Buteyko breathing techniques in asthma. *Med J Aust* 1998 Dec 7–12;169(11–12):575–8— available at   www.mja.com.au/public/issues/xmas98/bowler/ bowler.html.

p. 149   Opat AJ and others, A clinical trial of the Buteyko breathing technique in asthma as taught by a video, *J Asthma* 2000;37(7): 557–64.

p. 150   Ameisen PJ, *Every breath you take*, Landsdowne, Sydney, 1997.

p. 152   Weiner JM and Burdon JGW, Severe allergen-induced asthma despite the use of Buteyko breathing technique, *Med J Aust* 1999;171:109.

17 Which foods affect your asthma?

pp. 158–59   The elimination diet from the Royal Prince Alfred Hospital—see Clarke, p. 281, diet booklets, p. 300.

18 How to start the failsafe diet

p. 174   Fish oils—Mihrshahi S and others, The Childhood Asthma Prevention Study, *Control Clin Trials* 2001;22:333–54.

p. 175   Additives and immunosuppression—Ustyugova IV and others, Nitrates/nitrites alter human lymphocyte proliferation and cytokine production, *Arch Environ Contam Toxicol* 2002;43(3):270–6; Wajner M and others, Inhibition of mitogen-activated proliferation of human peripheral lymphocytes in vitro by propionic acid, *Clin Sci (Lond)* 1999 Jan;96(1):99–103.

p. 177   Ziem G and McTamney J, Profile of patients with chemical injury and sensitivity, *Environ Health Perspect*, 1997;105(Suppl 2): 2417–36.

p. 181   Policy statement: *Children, Adolescents and Television*, American Academy of Pediatrics, October 1995.

p. 184   Eskenazi B and others, Exposures of children to organophosphate pesticides and their potential adverse health effects, *Environ Health Perspect* 1999;107(Suppl 3):409–19.

19 How to avoid your problem foods

p. 187   Sulphites in more than half the foods tested—1994 Market Basket survey, see Notes for Chapter 2.

pp. 188–89   Sulphites in Australian foods—from the Australian Food Standards Code, www.foodstandards.com.au.

p. 190   Sulphites in US foods—Fazio T and Warner CR, A review of sulphites in foods, *Food Addit Contam* 1990;7(4):433–54.

p. 198   Annatto—Mikkelsen, see Notes for Chapter 4.

p. 202   Nitrates—*Additive Code Breaker*, see Notes for Chapter 9.

p. 209   Gluten—Palosuo K and others, A novel wheat gliadin as a cause of exercise-induced anaphylaxis, *J Allergy Clin Immunol* 1999;103(5 Pt 1):912–7.

20 Managing other asthma triggers

p. 211   Survey of triggers—Lewis J, Incidence and severity of asthma in the Greater Darwin area, Asthma Foundation of the Northern Territory, 1992.

p. 211   Laughter is a major asthma trigger, *New Scientist*, 28/3/02.

pp. 212–13   Werner D, *Where there is no doctor: a village health care handbook*, MacMillan assisted by Oxfam, many editions.

p. 215   Suphioglu C, Thunderstorm asthma due to grass pollen, *Int Arch Allergy Immunol* 1998;116(4):253–60.

p. 217   Thickett KM and others, Occupational asthma caused by chloramines in indoor swimming-pool air, *Eur Respir J* 2002;19(5): 827–32.

p. 218   Asthma from perfumes and other chemicals—Anderson RC and Anderson PJ, Acute toxic effects of fragrances, *Arch Environ Health* 1998;53(2):138–46; Pesticides and asthma—Eskanazi, see Notes for Chapter 18.

23 Food additives by code numbers

pp. 261–72   Colours, benzoates, sulphites, nitrates/nitrites, antioxidants, carrageenan, humectants—*Additive Code Breaker*, see Notes for Chapter 9.

p. 261   Cochineal—Chung K and others, Identification of carmine allergens among three carmine allergy patients, *Allergy* 2001;56(1): 73–7; Tanaka T, Reproductive and neurobehavioral effects of cochineal administered to mice in the diet, *Toxicol Ind Health*, 1995;11(1): 1–12.

p. 263   Canthaxanthin—Cortin P and others, Retinopathy due to canthazanthine, *Can J Ophthalmol* 1984;19(5):215–9.

p. 264   Sorbates—Swain AR and others, Royal Prince Alfred Hospital Allergy Unit, *Friendly Food*, Murdoch Books, 1991, Sydney.

p. 265   Propionates—Dengate and Ruben, see Notes for Chapter 5.

p. 268   Carrageenan—Tobacman JK, Review of harmful gastrointestinal effects of carrageenan in animal experiments, *Environ Health Perspect* 2001;109(10):983–94.

p. 270   MSG, see notes for Chapter 6 and also eye damage—Ohguro and others, A high dietary intake of sodium glutamate as flavoring (ajinomoto) causes gross changes in retinal morphology and function, *Exp Eye Res* 2002; 75(3):307–15; fibromyalgia—Smith JD and others, Relief of fibromyalgia symptoms following discontinuation of dietary excitotoxins, *Ann Pharmacother* 2001; headaches—Scopp AL, MSG and hydrolyzed vegetable protein induced headache, *Headache* 1991;31(2):107–10;;35(6):702–6; skin rash—Botey J and others, Monosodium glutamate and skin pathology in pediatric allergology, *Allergol Immunopathol (Madr)* 1988;16(6): 425–8; and burning, pressure, tightness or numbness in the face, neck, and upper chest—Settipane GA, The restaurant syndromes, *N Engl Reg Allergy Proc* 1987;8(1):39–46.

p. 271   Aspartame—Olney JW and others, Increasing brain tumor rates: is there a link to aspartame? *J Neuropathol Exp Neurol* 1996 Nov;55(11): 1115–23.

Support and further information

The Food Intolerance Network, PO Box 85, Parap, Northern Territory 0804, sdengate@ozemail.com.au, www.fedupwith foodadditives.info, provides:
- failsafe email newsletters
- failsafe discussion groups
- failsafe support groups

Adelaide, Liz, 08 8568 5040 •
Auckland NZ, Linda, 416 9438 •
Brisbane, Jan, 07 3264 4265 •
Canberra, Sheryl, 02 6294 1720 •

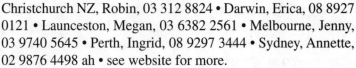

Christchurch NZ, Robin, 03 312 8824 • Darwin, Erica, 08 8927 0121 • Launceston, Megan, 03 6382 2561 • Melbourne, Jenny, 03 9740 5645 • Perth, Ingrid, 08 9297 3444 • Sydney, Annette, 02 9876 4498 ah • see website for more.

Asthma Foundations, freecall 1800 645 130 bh, www.asthma australia.org.au • Adelaide 08 8362 6272 • Brisbane 07 3252 7677 • Darwin 08 8922 8817 • Hobart 03 6223 7725 • Melbourne 03 9326 7088 • Perth 08 9481 1234 • Sydney 02 9906 3233.

Books, booklets and videos
The Failsafe Cookbook, by Sue Dengate, Random House, 2001 contains failsafe recipes and suggestions for every occasion.
Fed Up by Sue Dengate, Random House, 1998 details how food can affect children's health, learning ability and behaviour.
The Simplified Elimination Diet and *Salicylates, Amines and MSG*, are available as a set of two booklets from your dietitian or from the Royal Prince Alfred Hospital Allergy Unit at $7 a set. Ask for an order form or send your money with your

name and address and the name and address of your doctor. Booklets will be sent to your doctor. The RPAH's cookbook, *Friendly Food* by Drs Swain and others, Murdoch Books, 1991, is also available: RPAH Allergy Unit, Suite 210, 100 Carillon Avenue, Newtown NSW 2042, (allergy@email.cs.nsw.gov.au). The failsafe diet is based on the on-going research of Dr Anne Swain, Dr Velencia Soutter and Dr Robert Loblay of the Allergy Unit. This group and their publications act as a resource to dietitians around the world.

New Additive Code Breaker by Maurice Hanssen, Lothian, 1996.

Fast Food Nation by Eric Schlosser, Penguin, 2001—a gripping read.

Allergyfree Gardening by T. Ogren, Ten Speed Press, 2001, www.allergyfree-gardening.com.

Raising healthy children in a toxic world, Landrigan, PJ and others, Rodale, 2001, a practical book by leading researchers.

Asthma management handbook, National Asthma Council: www.NationalAsthma.org.au.

1–2–3 Magic is an expensive but effective US behaviour management video available from www.amazon.com or see Triple P below.

The Explosive Child by Ross W Greene, Harper Collins, New York, 2001, www.explosivechild.com.

Breathing Works for Asthma by Dinah Bradley and Tania Clifton-Smith, Tandem Press, NZ 2002, www.breathing works.com.

Websites

Allergy and anaphylaxis: www.allergyfacts.com.au.

Australian Breastfeeding Association: www.breastfeeding.asn.au.

Buteyko Breathing Method, freecall in Australia 1800 658 818, www.buteykovideo.com and www.buteyko.com.au.

Centre for Children's Health and the Environment, www.childenvironment.org.

Centre for Science in the Public Interest: www.cspinet.org.

Dairy free capsules with Lactobacillus GG—www.culturelle.com.

Food additives:
  sulphites: http://members@aol.com/nosulfites.
  MSG: www.truthinlabeling.org.
  tartrazine: http://tartrazine.tripod.com/.

How to avoid harmful chemicals: www.checnet.org.

Prescription drugs: www.myDr.com.au, www.my.webMD.com.

Public Citizen health research group for drugs, www.citizen.org/hrg.

This pharmacy sells failsafe vitamin supplements: www.pharmacydirect.com.au.

Triple P Parenting course: www.triplep.net.

Petitions

- *To ban tartrazine* (102, yellow #5), send an email *to*: fdadockets@oc.fda.gov. *Subject line*: Docket #02P-0345, Delist Yellow #5; *Message*: I vote to ban Yellow #5. Give your name, address and phone number. *Optional*: give a reason.

- *To ban* the use of calcium propionate, 282, and sodium metabisulphite, 223, in bread, visit your nearest Brumby's store and sign their petition sheet.

Index

Also published by Random House Australia

The Failsafe Cookbook
Reducing food chemicals for calm, happy families
Sue Dengate

Sue Dengate's revolutionary cookbook is an essential tool for parents wanting a calmer, happier—and healthier—family. Her bestselling book *Fed Up* opened the eyes of thousands of desperate parents to the adverse effects of synthetic additives and natural chemicals in foods.

Based on groundbreaking research, *Fed Up* showed how learning difficulties, behavioural problems and minor chronic illnesses in children and adults can all be the result of intolerances to food chemicals.

In her comprehensive *Failsafe Cookbook*, Sue has written and compiled hundreds of new and improved recipes for all kinds of occasions, as well as detailed information about food intolerance and the elimination diet.

With the help of these tasty and easy-to-follow recipes for breakfasts, lunches, main meals and desserts, through to food for special occasions, vegetarian cooking and gluten-free food—and by following Sue's step-by-step guide to the elimination diet—it is possible to free of a wide range of health and behavioural problems.

Fed Up
How food affects your child and what you can do about it
Sue Dengate

Fed Up is Sue Dengate's bestselling, meticulously researched response to the wide-ranging problems of food intolerance and how it affects people, from learning difficulties to behavioural problems and minor chronic illness. This handbook is an essential tool for childrearing and an indispensable guide for adults.

You would think that …

Fruit is the healthiest food.
Wrong. Fruit can be as bad as additives for some children.

Kids are just like that.
Wrong. Added and natural food chemicals can cause:
• irritability, restlessness, a 'short fuse' when things go wrong
• poor reading or school performance
• 'restless legs', slow to fall asleep or night-waking
• headaches or stomach aches
• itchy skin rashes or bedwetting
• disorganisation, lack of energy
• some symptoms of ADHD and oppositional defiant disorder
• frequent ear infections, asthma, stuffy or runny nose

Reactions to food addtives are quick and easy to identify
Wrong. Most reactions are delayed.

Food additives would be banned if they were harmful
Wrong. Food additives are not tested for effects on behaviour or learning.

Praise for Fed Up

'A reminder to all parents to take a closer look at what their children are eating'
Melbourne Age